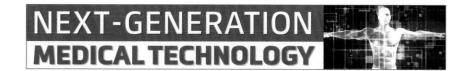

NEXT-GENERATION
MEDICAL TECHNOLOGY

Virtual Reality and Medicine

Other titles in the *Next-Generation Medical Technology* series include:

Genetics and Medicine

Nanotechnology and Medicine

Robotics and Medicine

3D Printing and Medicine

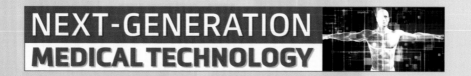

Virtual Reality and Medicine

James Roland

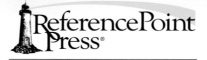

ReferencePoint Press®

San Diego, CA

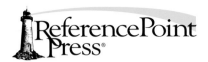

© 2018 ReferencePoint Press, Inc.
Printed in the United States

For more information, contact:
ReferencePoint Press, Inc.
PO Box 27779
San Diego, CA 92198
www.ReferencePointPress.com

LIBRARY OF CONGRESS CATALOGING-IN-PUBLICATION DATA

Name: Roland, James, author.
Title: Virtual Reality and Medicine/by James Roland.
Description: San Diego, CA: ReferencePoint Press, Inc., 2018. | Series:
Next-Generation Medical Technology series | Audience: Grade 9 to 12. | Includes
    bibliographical references and index.
Identifiers: LCCN 2017041158 (print) | LCCN 2017045826 (ebook) | ISBN 9781682823347 (eBook)
    | ISBN 9781682823330 (hardback)
Subjects: LCSH: Virtual reality in medicine. | Computer vision in medicine.
Classification: LCC R859.7.C67 (ebook) | LCC R859.7.C67 R65 2018 (print) | DDC 610.285—dc23
LC record available at https://lccn.loc.gov/2017041158

CONTENTS

IMPORTANT EVENTS IN THE HISTORY OF VIRTUAL REALITY

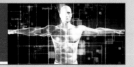

1935
Science fiction writer Stanley Weinbaum publishes "Pygmalion's Spectacles," a story in which characters wear special goggles that allow them to see, feel, hear, and touch life in a fictional world.

1793
Robert Barker displays his 360-degree panoramic painting of the Edinburgh skyline, considered one of the earliest attempts to immerse an audience in a work of art.

1939
The View-Master, a stereoscope-like toy for children, hits the market.

1969
Myron Krueger coins the term *artificial reality* to describe his computer-generated environments that respond to the characters in those environments.

1800 / **1940** **1950** **1960** **1970**

1838
Charles Wheatstone invents the stereoscope, a device that uses special lenses to view two similar images placed side by side to give the appearance of three dimensions.

1960
Cinematographer Morton Heilig patents the Telesphere Mask, the first head-mounted display (HMD) used to watch movies in 3-D and with stereo sound.

1962
Morton Heilig patents Sensorama, a film-viewing immersive experience that featured a vibrating seat and piped-in scents and wind to enhance the on-screen action.

1968
Inventor Ivan Sutherland creates the Sword of Damocles, the first virtual reality/augmented reality headset linked to a computer rather than a camera.

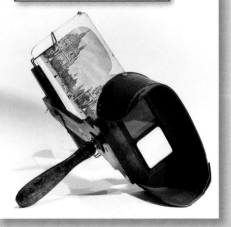

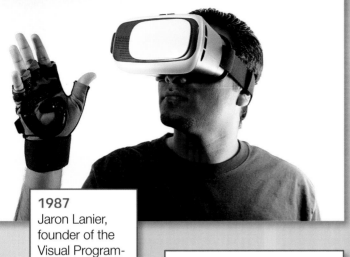

2015
Western University of Health Sciences in California opens the first medical school VR learning center in the United States.

2016
Dr. Shafi Ahmed performs a cancer surgery that is broadcast around the world in VR.

1987
Jaron Lanier, founder of the Visual Programming Lab, coins the term *virtual reality*. The company sells the first commercial virtual reality (VR) goggles and gloves.

2008
Results of a clinical trial of Virtual Iraq, a VR simulation to treat veterans dealing with post-traumatic stress disorder, show significant improvement in how the vets cope with their stress.

2017
University of California–San Diego opens the first VR lab for undergraduates in a US university.

1980   **1990**   **2000**   **2010**   **2020**

1982
Thomas Furness develops the Visually Coupled Airborne Systems Simulator, an advanced flight simulator in which the pilot wears an HMD.

1996
Max North, a pioneer in VR therapy, publishes the first book on the subject, *Virtual Reality Therapy: An Innovative Paradigm*.

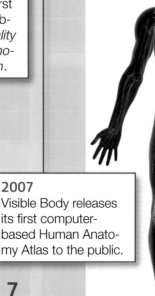

2007
Visible Body releases its first computer-based Human Anatomy Atlas to the public.

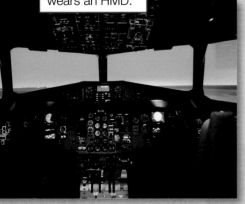

7

Virtual Reality Transforms Medicine

On April 14, 2016, a cancer surgeon in London, England, performed a first-of-its-kind operation. There was nothing particularly fascinating about the procedure itself. The patient was a man in his seventies having a cancerous tumor removed from his colon. What made this operation so groundbreaking was who could observe it—and *how* they could watch every move the doctors and nurses made.

That operation in Royal London Hospital was performed by Dr. Shafi Ahmed, and it was broadcast live through virtual reality (VR). Anyone around the world with VR headsets and the right app for their smartphones or who went to the Medical Realities website (Ahmed's VR-based medical training company) could see exactly what Ahmed was seeing. And because the operation was filmed with two 360-degree cameras with multiple lenses, viewers could walk around the operating room to get other angles on the surgery. Virtual reality (and the related technology of augmented reality, or AR) are likely to advance doctor training and the practice of medicine in ways that, for now, still can only be imagined. "I believe that virtual reality and augmented reality can revolutionize surgical education and training, particularly for developing countries that don't have the resources and facilities of NHS [England's National Health Service] hospitals," says Ahmed. "I am very excited about the expansion of this program to bring more medical learning to the world."[1]

Playing Tricks on the Mind

Virtual reality as people know it today is basically computer technology tricking the brain into believing it is in the environment that is created with sights and sounds and delivered through a sophisticated headset. The goggles in the headset deliver three-dimensional images that fill a person's field of vision—the entire area that can be seen in whatever direction the eyes are facing. Many VR devices include sound effects pumped through headphones that block out other noise. Some systems use gloves fitted with sensors. These are called haptic systems. In simple terms, VR technology includes trackers in the headset, gloves, handheld controller, or even a suit in very sophisticated systems. The trackers detect the movement and position of the user and signal the headset computer to reflect that information in the environment seen by the user in his or her goggles. As the VR user moves and looks around in real space, the point of view and action in the virtual space moves and changes accordingly.

augmented

added to something to make it bigger or greater

To most people, virtual reality technology is little more than a way to add a three-dimensional environment to video games or to put viewers closer than ever to the action in a movie. But this rapidly improving technology is revolutionizing medicine, too. Medical students learn anatomy in 3-D using VR equipment instead of human cadavers. Athletes recover from injuries with VR's help. Surgeons and surgical patients use VR to preview their operations before going through the real thing. And hospital patients are using VR to distract them from pain or the monotony of extended bed rest. And what is most exciting is that the role VR will play in medicine is only just now being developed.

haptic

relating to the sense of touch, particularly in the perception and manipulation of objects

VR certainly did not start out as a tool to help make medical miracles happen. Virtual reality as it is known today was part of the computer revolution of the 1980s. But its original roots go back centuries to an era when artists painted huge panoramas that were displayed in circular buildings. Visitors stood in the middle of these rotundas to take in the 360-degree artwork of a skyline of a faraway city or the cannons, horses, and swordsmen in a battle waged long ago. The efforts to transport audiences to a different time and place got more technologically sophisticated through the years. As computer technology raced along at the end of the twentieth century and the beginning of the twenty-first century, inventors and doctors like Ahmed saw the potential of VR not just for entertainment but for medical education and treatment.

Twenty-First-Century Anatomy Lessons

Medical colleges now use a variety of VR and non-VR simulations to enhance the teaching of anatomy and surgical procedures. Case Western Reserve University School of Medicine in Cleveland, Ohio, has replaced its cadaver lab with VR headsets and other teaching tools that make it possible for students to rotate a virtual body and explore the various layers of skin, muscle, and tissue with a sensor probe rather than a scalpel. The simulated body can be manipulated to show the effects of many different diseases and injuries that would not be visible in a cadaver. Additionally, VR simulations avoid the problem of degraded organs or tissue, a condition that frequently occurs with cadavers.

VR is not taking the place of all hands-on training with real patients, but it is playing a bigger role in the education and clinical

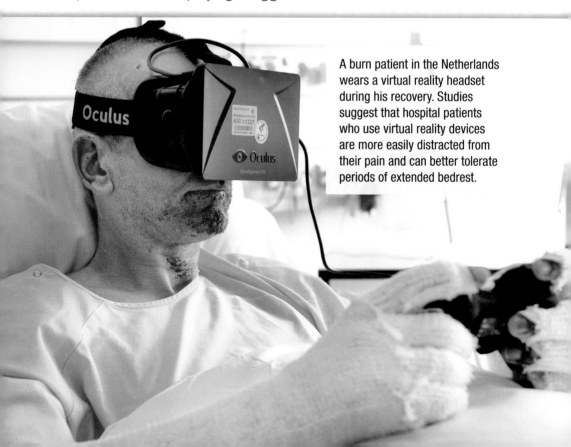

A burn patient in the Netherlands wears a virtual reality headset during his recovery. Studies suggest that hospital patients who use virtual reality devices are more easily distracted from their pain and can better tolerate periods of extended bedrest.

practice of a new generation of physicians. In some cases it is the patient who wears the VR headset during a procedure. Neurosurgeons are using VR to help see how the brain reacts during brain surgery. A VR program can trigger a conscious patient's brain to respond to certain stimuli, allowing the neurosurgeon to see immediately if the procedure is working. The brain's psychological and emotional elements also benefit from VR-based therapy. The technology helps people deal with phobias such as fear of flying or with post-traumatic stress disorder (PTSD) by placing them in safe situations that allow the individual to confront a fear or anxiety in a controlled environment with a therapist close by.

Patients are using VR for a wide range of other purposes, too. For example, a Boston hospital takes patients through a VR program that lets them see the operating room where they will have surgery, shows them the equipment, and even lets them "meet" some of the people who will be part of their surgical and postsurgical care. The idea is that by letting a patient have a virtual surgical experience, he or she will feel less anxiety about the actual operation. VR headsets are also given to patients as an escape from long days and nights in a hospital bed. VR games and travel tours are proving to be effective distractions.

VR does not just help take people into new places virtually; the technology is also literally helping patients with brain injuries or who have lost a leg get from one place to another. Treatment that combines physical therapy with VR has stroke survivors moving across the room, down the hall, and toward a more mobile future than they might have imagined. Amputees are recovering using VR technology's ability to provide a virtual limb to temporarily replace the lost one.

The future of VR and medicine is being programmed right now, but this technology is already being used in some mind-blowing ways to help doctors and their patients. In the summer of 2017, for example, surgeons used VR technology to successfully separate conjoined infants in Minnesota. "The medical uses are pretty amazing," says Tony Parisi, who oversees VR development at Unity Technologies, a video game company that is moving rapidly into developing medical VR applications. "We're seeing the perfect confluence. Anything you can do to train people more quickly, effectively, and cheaply is a boon to the healthcare industry. VR is a rapidly evolving technology that solves a lot of problems here."[2]

CHAPTER 1

A History of Illusion

Virtual reality today conjures up computer-generated images that offer passage to a three-dimensional fictional world for someone wearing special goggles or a headset. VR can also take users on virtual vacations to exotic locations around the real world. And this swiftly changing technology enables people to venture into places they could never hope to go: inside the human brain, heart, ear, and other locations within the body.

Doctors and computer engineers are working together to create virtual reality mechanisms to solve real-world medical challenges, but this is not where the technology began. The roots of virtual reality lie in oil paintings, not pixels—the tiny illuminated areas on a computer screen that combine to form recognizable images. Artists have been trying for centuries to transport their audiences to faraway places and exciting events without asking them to leave an auditorium or gallery.

Panoramic Paintings

In 1787 an Irish artist named Robert Barker patented plans for a round building to be constructed in Leicester Square, a wealthy commercial section in West London. His building was to surround a huge circular painting Barker had done of Edinburgh, Scotland. Visitors to *The Panorama* paid one shilling (a lot of money at the time) to stand in a rotunda lighted in just the right way to give the cityscape a more lifelike feel. Viewers gazed at the 360-degree work of art, one of the earliest attempts at virtual reality.

In the century that followed Barker's breakthrough, panoramic paintings that immersed viewers in the subject matter captured the imaginations of people around the world. One of the most popular subjects of these circular masterpieces was warfare. In one direction, a viewer could see a general leading his troops on horseback, while on the other side of the room, the enemy approached with swords glistening and horses frothing.

panorama

a picture that contains a wide, unbroken view of a place or event that surrounds the viewer

Stereoscopic Vision

It was not long before some innovative tinkerers and artists realized that lenses, such as those used in eyeglasses or telescopes, could be manipulated to present an even greater sense of immersion in a scene. One of the first visionary VR inventors was English scientist Charles Wheatstone, who developed the first stereoscope in 1838. Wheatstone discovered that each eye sends a slightly different two-dimensional image of an object to the brain. The brain then combines those two images into a single three-dimensional image. With that in mind, Wheatstone invented a device in which two nearly identical images viewed side by side gave the images depth—the way people view 3-D movies today. The early devices were relatively simple. Two separate lenses were fitted into a small box about 2 inches (5cm) apart. Slits in the box were made to control the amount of light that entered. Another opening allowed the pictures to be placed into the back of the box. The user looked with both eyes at the side-by-side images, and the brain did the rest, processing the two pictures as one scene with three dimensions, not just a flat two-dimensional rendering.

stereoscope

a lensed device in which two photographs taken at slightly different angles are placed next to each other to give the illusion of depth

Wheatstone's stereoscope led to the development of other similar devices, such as the popular children's View-Master stereoscope in 1939. The View-Master marked a big improvement over the old-fashioned stereoscopes. Specifically, older stereoscopes

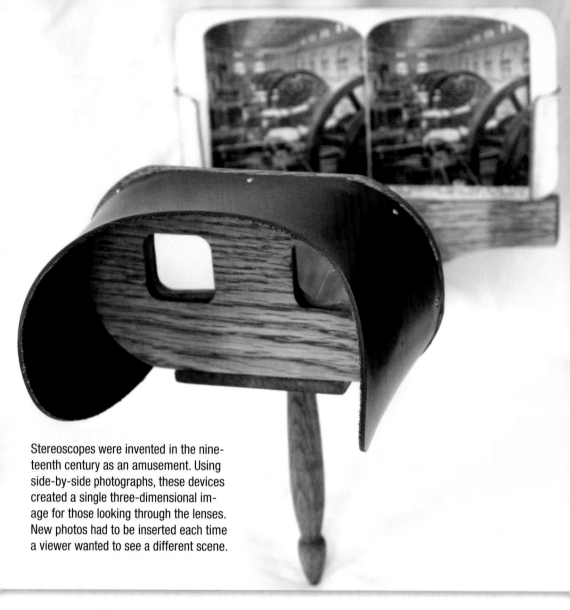

Stereoscopes were invented in the nineteenth century as an amusement. Using side-by-side photographs, these devices created a single three-dimensional image for those looking through the lenses. New photos had to be inserted each time a viewer wanted to see a different scene.

could only hold one image at a time. To see more than one scene the user had to take out the pictures and put a new set in each time. With a View-Master, they could see seven images per reel, the round card that contained tiny pictures around its edges that were magnified by the lenses in the toy.

With the View-Master still a big hit with kids in the 1950s, the next step was to make moving pictures part of the VR experience. The man who pioneered that effort and who could rightly wear the crown as the Father of Virtual Reality was Morton Heilig. He was a California cinematographer who had an idea for expanding what movie audiences could see and experience compared with what they view in a traditional movie theater. After years of trial and error, in 1962 he built Sensorama, a viewing system that included a seat and a metal hood that users looked under to watch the films Heilig made. They were short films, such as *Motorcycle*, which took viewers on a 3-D motorcycle ride through Brooklyn—complete with a vibrating seat, a breeze in the face, and smells of the city. Sensorama films and the viewing equipment were expensive, and Heilig failed to draw investors to his early VR effort. The same had been true of Heilig's earlier invention—a head-mounted film display system called the Telesphere Mask, introduced in 1960. The bulky goggles featured stereoscopic 3-D and wide-vision viewing. Wide-vision viewing is possible when lenses are curved to expand the field of vision from what a person would normally have without any special goggles. This is similar to a wide-angle camera lens or backup camera in a car that expands what can be seen through normal peripheral vision. What the Telesphere Mask lacked was motion tracking—a key feature of modern VR goggles.

Motion tracking means the movements of the VR user are represented in the action on-screen. Some VR systems have gloves that allow a player to squeeze his or her trigger finger to fire a gun in a VR game. Other, more complex systems have lasers crisscrossing the room where the VR user is playing a game. The player's movements, such as running or jumping, are duplicated on-screen with a minimal delay. Many systems have only head-tracking technology, so as a user looks to the right, the action on the screen will swing right also. One of the earliest head-mounted displays (HMDs, or the goggles and headsets that are standard in VR) that included motion tracking was developed in 1961 by engineers with Philco. The system was actually designed for military purposes. A soldier could wear an HMD that was linked to a remote closed-circuit camera set up to look out for the enemy. As the soldier turned to the right or left, the camera in another location would turn also. The Headsight, as it was called, and other early HMDs did not have anything like the computer technology VR headsets have today. But they were among the first devices to preview what was ahead for VR.

Computer Tech Meets VR Vision

By the middle of the 1960s, the possibilities of virtual reality captured the imagination of many in the computer world. Computer scientist Ivan Sutherland, an early pioneer in computer graphics and the Internet, wrote a paper in 1965 about the "ultimate display," in which people could interact with a computer-generated virtual world in the same way they do with the real world. He wrote:

> The ultimate display would, of course, be a room within which the computer can control the existence of matter. A chair displayed in such a room would be good enough to sit in. Handcuffs displayed in such a room would be confining, and a bullet displayed in such a room would be fatal. With appropriate programming such a display could literally be the Wonderland into which Alice walked.[3]

Though VR technology has not yet fulfilled Sutherland's prediction, advances in virtual reality moved rapidly starting in the late 1960s. In 1969, for instance, computer engineers started using the term *artificial reality* to describe their simulated environments. Computer artist Myron Krueger coined the term to describe computer-based games and art projects, in which the computer-generated environments responded to the characters' actions within those environments. These projects had names such as GLOWFLOW and PSYCHIC SPACE. In the 1970s Krueger's work eventually led to the creation of VIDEOPLACE, an artificial reality lab at the University of Connecticut. A network of cameras, projectors, and computers recorded the actions of people in different rooms within the lab. The video recordings of the people were projected as silhouettes on screens so that they appeared to interact with each other even though the participants themselves were in separate rooms and could not see each other. The effect was so startling for the participants that they would actually try to move out of the way if they saw that their own silhouette looked as though it would collide with another silhouette.

Then in 1987 computer scientist and artist Jaron Lanier coined the term *virtual reality* while developing some of the world's first multiperson virtual worlds and avatars (characters representing people in video games, Internet forums, and so on). He had recently founded VPL Research, which was the first business to

Who Is Jaron Lanier?

Jaron Lanier is credited with popularizing the term *virtual reality*. The former game designer left the video game company Atari to launch VPL Research in 1985. *VPL* stood for "Visual Programming Languages." It was the first company to sell VR goggles and gloves. Though Lanier's company filed for bankruptcy in 1999, he remains a pivotal figure in the history of VR. Born in New York City in 1960 but raised in New Mexico, Lanier persuaded New Mexico State University to let him enroll at age thirteen. This brilliant young man eventually took graduate-level courses and earned a National Science Foundation grant to study mathematical notation—a writing system that uses symbols to represent mathematic concepts. This led him to learn computer programming, and that drew him to Santa Cruz, California, at the start of the personal computer era in the early 1980s. Lanier is also a visual artist, musician, composer, and writer. He has written books about how humans can and should interact with technology, including 2013's award-winning *Who Owns the Future?* Lanier has worked for several tech companies, been a visiting scholar, and has continued to be a virtual reality innovator, most recently at Microsoft.

market VR goggles and gloves. Among VPL's products were the Dataglove and the EyePhone. The Dataglove was one of the first wired gloves, which are now standard VR equipment. It is a glove that allows the user to manipulate things in a VR environment by moving their hand and fingers. The EyePhone was an early example of the VR headsets in use today. Lanier's inventions and those of other innovators in the 1980s and 1990s inspired other creative computer scientists' greater interest in the potential of VR for entertainment and other purposes.

From then on, VR research and products became more widely known, and before long, VR went mainstream with arcade games and products kids and adults could use at home. Video game makers Sega and Nintendo came out with VR game systems in the 1990s.

Beyond Fun and Games

But it was not until the 1990s that scientists and engineers in a broader range of fields began seeing how VR could enhance their work. One of the first uses of virtual reality in medicine was for teaching anatomy. Virtual reality was also used to instruct students in basic medical and dental procedures such as tooth extractions or lumbar punctures (which involve a needle withdrawing a small sample of spinal fluid from the lower back). As with many computer-related innovations, these first medical applications were hit-or-miss. The relatively poor or simple graphics were not especially helpful to students and surgeons. But

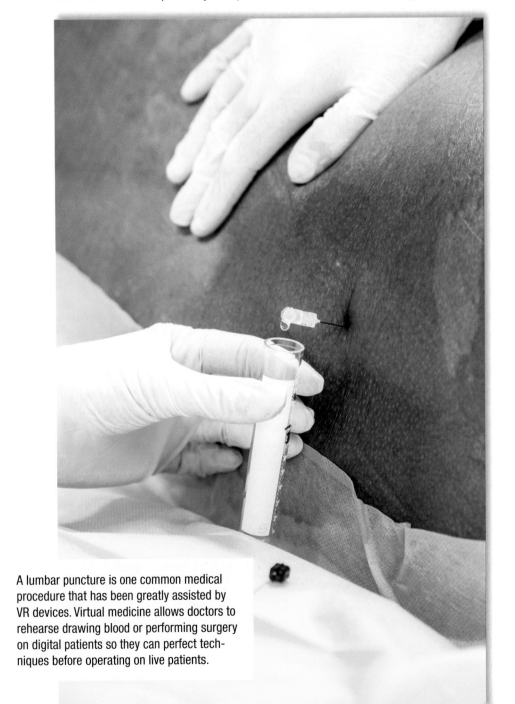

A lumbar puncture is one common medical procedure that has been greatly assisted by VR devices. Virtual medicine allows doctors to rehearse drawing blood or performing surgery on digital patients so they can perfect techniques before operating on live patients.

gradually, the image details improved. Both students and surgeons could practice procedures on virtual patients without fear of harm. Virtual reality also enhanced a doctor's ability to diagnose medical conditions. Virtual patients can be given all sorts of diseases and injuries—and the symptoms that go with them. This allows medical students to become familiar with common conditions and their symptoms, which can be helpful in making diagnoses in the real world.

Many other types of computer-generated simulations are assisting health care students and providers around the world. A VR company called Geomagic, which started in the 1990s as Sensable, was at the forefront of haptic feedback in medical training. Haptic feedback is the sensation of force, vibration, or motion that a VR system or other computer-based piece of technology sends back to the user. A smartphone that vibrates when using a navigation app, for example, is using haptic feedback. Sensable's engineers re-created the "force feedback" a doctor gets when a medical instrument touches an organ or bone. A device attached by a robotic arm to the computer and monitor is fitted with a special stylus that can be used like a virtual scalpel or probe. When it looks as though the probe is touching a skull on-screen, for instance, the user feels a simulated version of the hard bones of the cranium through the robotic arm and stylus. Haptic feedback adds another layer of realism to medical training on simulated patients.

force feedback

the sensation of touching something solid or forceful that users experience in some VR environments

Many Possibilities

One of the most inspiring aspects of VR in health care is the willingness of hospitals, universities, and other entities to share their work and to expand the reach of this new technology. The University of Illinois–Chicago, which created one of the first university-based VR medical labs in the country, used a National Institutes of Health grant to build computer-generated models of an inner ear, heart, pelvis, and other body parts. The models were then

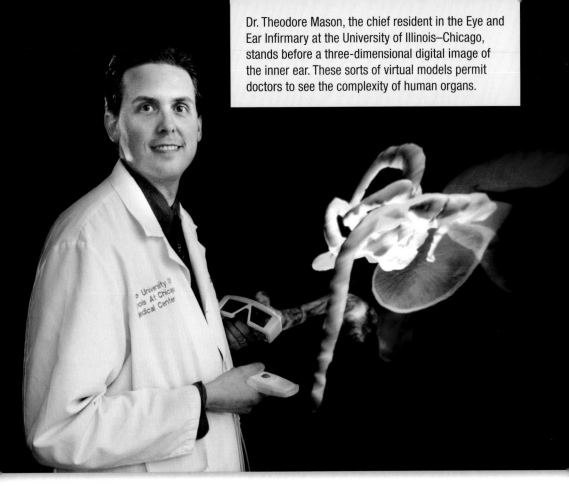

Dr. Theodore Mason, the chief resident in the Eye and Ear Infirmary at the University of Illinois–Chicago, stands before a three-dimensional digital image of the inner ear. These sorts of virtual models permit doctors to see the complexity of human organs.

shared with other institutions. Dr. Theodore Mason, chief resident in the Eye and Ear Infirmary at the university, and others in the medical VR field realized early on that it would be a great advantage for a surgeon to perform a virtual operation prior to using a scalpel on an actual patient. During a grand opening tour of the lab in 2000, Mason pointed out the educational value of a 3-D VR simulation of the inner ear. "If a picture's worth a thousand words, then a model like this is worth a thousand pictures,"[4] he said.

The value of VR in medicine is even greater to young doctors without access to top surgeons and the best facilities. They can, in effect, "catch up" with their peers with increasingly sophisticated VR medical technology. Shafi Ahmed, the London surgeon who performed the first operation broadcast in VR, predicts virtual reality and other advances in computers and communication will transform medicine around the world. Says Ahmed:

Imagine that you're a surgical trainee in Tanzania. You're restrained by geography, you're in a rural setting, but you want some training. You want to improve the standards of your health care system, as every doctor does. . . . Imagine you're a surgeon, maybe an attending in Bangladesh, a population of 150 million with a very poor infrastructure of training and teaching. . . . Imagine you're a school kid in an inner city area, a poor district. But then you want to be a surgeon, you want to train to be a medic, you want to access information. You'd like to know what it's like and immerse yourself.[5]

But not all fascinating advances are happening on the surgery side. In 2014 at Boston's Beth Israel Deaconess Medical Center, doctors started experimenting with Google Glass to access information on their glasses while they were working with patients. Google Glass, introduced by Google in 2014, is a head-mounted optical display that looks like eyeglasses. The original version, in which consumers could check Facebook, the news, and use other apps, flopped within a couple of years. In the summer of 2017, Alphabet (Google's parent company) introduced Glass Enterprise Edition for the workplace. People working in hospitals, factories, and other locations could use Google Glass to look up instructions, checklists, and other work-related information. In a medical setting, the goal of Google Glass–like applications for doctors and nurses is to provide real-time access to patient records and other vital information in a secure manner—all hands free. "I believe wearable computing will replace tablet-based computing for many clinicians who need their hands free and instant access to information,"[6] says Dr. John Halamka, chief information officer of the hospital.

Future Role

VR's rapid ascent in medicine shows no signs of slowing. Creative thinkers in the medical and computer fields are developing new applications for VR and AR. And it is proving to be profitable, too. In 2016 Oculus Rift VR headsets were first sold to the public. The maker, Oculus VR, had started out as a Kickstarter campaign in 2012. Two years later, Facebook purchased Oculus for $2 billion—a sign that virtual reality was also a commercial reality. Oculus Rift technology became the centerpiece of many nonentertainment VR efforts in science, engineering, and medicine.

Sizable financial investment in medical VR can be found everywhere. In 2017 the University of Nebraska Medical Center (UNMC) in Omaha broke ground on a $118.9 million, 191,884-square-foot (17,827 sq. m) facility that will use AR and VR to train the doctors, nurses, and other health care providers of the future. "Learners do best by having experience, whether it's learning how to play a sport, a musical instrument or, in my case, do cardiac surgery. The more experience, the more practice, the more hands-on opportunities we get the better off we are to deliver high quality, safe, effective and patient-centered care," says Dr. Jeffrey Gold, chancellor of UNMC. He believes virtual reality technology will

Enhancing STEM Education with Virtual Reality

Even before students arrive at med school, they are becoming well versed in how VR can take their learning to previously unimagined levels. As schools around the world are boosting their STEM programs, educators are finding exciting opportunities for VR in the classroom. A well-equipped STEM lab has electrical circuits and computers, equipment for physics experiments, and materials for robotics and other engineering projects. But a virtual STEM lab can eliminate the need for much of that equipment, reducing the burden on schools to come up with the space and money for exciting STEM projects. For example, at Meads Middle School in Northville, Michigan, technology teacher Tonya Nugent takes her students through a VR experience in which the students design floor plans for restaurants of their own creation. "Students use the design process commonly found in engineering to create an example drawing of their floor plan from a bird's-eye view or top-down perspective," Nugent says. "Many had a greater understanding of the design concept of a restaurant floor plan." Likewise, virtual chemistry experiments can be done without the risks associated with dangerous chemicals. Unimersiv, an educational VR company, also has programs that take students on virtual tours of the International Space Station, Stonehenge, and human anatomy. Teachers find their students are eager to don VR goggles in class and explore the world.

Quoted in Jennifer Zaino, "Promote STEM Learning Success with Virtual Reality in Education," Insights, May 3, 2017. https://insights.samsung.com.

provide more opportunities for medical students to repeat lessons and procedures far more times than would be possible in a traditional medical school environment. Students can work on many types of VR simulations on their own without having to be in a structured classroom or lab setting with a professor present.

VR's history and its exciting future in medicine represent a combined effort of computer scientists and visionaries who see the intersection of virtual and real worlds as a place where just about anything can happen. While no one can predict exactly what medicine will look like in the decades ahead, there is no doubt that VR will play an important role.

CHAPTER 2

Training Tool

Medical schools train future doctors in techniques for diagnosing and treating patients. For many years that training was based largely on textbooks and classroom lectures. Medical students also gained much of their knowledge of human anatomy by working on cadavers or by observing more experienced doctors performing, for instance, actual surgeries. While those staples of a doctor's education are still used today, computer technology and virtual reality are rapidly changing how the next generation of physicians and surgeons are learning their craft.

Digital Anatomy Class

Western University of Health Sciences in Pomona, California, was one of the first med schools in the world to create a VR facility for its students. Western's Virtual Reality Learning Center makes it possible for students to "lift" images, such as of a heart or brain, off a computer screen and manipulate them with a stylus as though the items were right in front of them in space. Among the tools used by students at the learning center are Oculus Rift VR goggles, iPads, and anatomical models that include organs made of synthetic but lifelike materials. At the center of the facility is the Anatomage Virtual Dissection Table. This amazing piece of technology uses diagnostic imaging tools such as computed tomography (CT) scans, magnetic

> **computed tomography**
>
> also called CT, a type of medical imaging that combines multiple layered images of a body structure to create a three-dimensional view

resonance imaging, digital photographs of cadavers, and X-rays to create multilayered, three-dimensional human models. Students stand around the table and examine organs, muscles, bones, and other features of human anatomy. The virtual bodies can be turned to give students a better view, and a stylus probe allows students to virtually separate layers of tissue to see how the body's systems work together or to look for tumors or other signs of disease.

Dentist Robert Hasel, associate dean of Western University's Simulation, Immersion, and Digital Learning, says the various features of the learning center complement each other in enhancing the students' understanding of anatomy, disease, and medicine. Hasel explains:

vasculature

the network of veins, arteries, and other blood vessels in the body

> We can remove and hold some of the organs that are molded and cast in silicone, similar to the texture and weight of actual organs. For example, the liver is made with a semi-transparent material that shows the lobes of liver, the vasculature and the ducts. The lungs are made out of light and spongy material. As you hold the lung in your hand, it builds a 3-D mental relationship in your mind to augment what you've seen on the Anatomage table and the iPad or textbook. By placing the stylus probe on certain structures, you can see how they relate to surrounding structures. For instance, you can look at which ribs are behind the lung tissue and where the kidneys are located in relation to the diaphragm, and at the same time see the cross-sections in three different planes.[7]

While Western was among the first to use this combination of technology, other medical schools around the world are turning to VR as a teaching tool. "The more these technologies are available, the more they will be accepted, and more software programs will be developed for use in the classroom," says Hasel. "It will take a while for these technologies and VR to be embraced on a wide scale by the academic community, but it will eventually

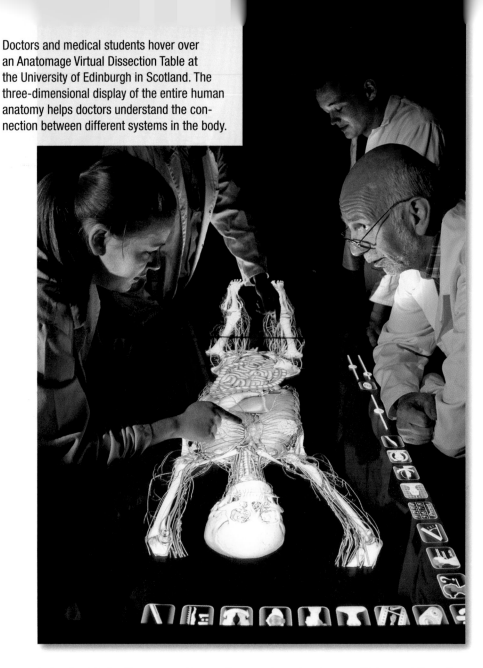

Doctors and medical students hover over an Anatomage Virtual Dissection Table at the University of Edinburgh in Scotland. The three-dimensional display of the entire human anatomy helps doctors understand the connection between different systems in the body.

take hold. In the meantime, the early adaptors will be setting the course and having all the fun."[8]

Better than Cadavers

One place VR has taken hold is Case Western Reserve University School of Medicine in Ohio. Like Western University in California, Case Western is using virtual reality technology to teach students about human anatomy. Case Western has turned to Microsoft's HoloLens system for this task. This system uses visual projections on top of the user's real-world view—a type of augmented reality. The HoloLens system allows students to explore skin layers, muscles, blood vessels, organs, and bones. Students can walk around the body or view a magnified, isolated organ such as the heart or the intricate network of arteries and veins that compose the circulatory system.

Case Western has embraced VR to the point that there is no longer a cadaver lab on campus. According to Mark Griswold, a professor in the Department of Radiology at Case Western:

> Obviously, this is a pretty big challenge. We've had many hundreds of years of teaching anatomy the same way, but we also thought the time was right to think about doing it in a new way. . . . It's very difficult to maintain a cadaver lab, the cost and infrastructure required to maintain that is very difficult. Not only is there the challenge of having people's bodies donated, but there's a lot of challenge around all the environmental concerns.[9]

Cadavers and donated organs are limited in their usefulness, whereas a computer-generated body or organ can be operated on countless times. A working eye and a beating heart are not available in a cadaver, and some body parts are simply difficult to comprehend, even with a cadaver. A University of Illinois–Chicago computer model allows students to practice delicate surgery on the retina—an opportunity that could only be possible in the virtual world. "It shows anatomic structures in a way that are otherwise impossible to see. You can't dissect a cadaver this way,"[10] says Dr. Jonathan Silverstein, a surgery professor and codirector of the university's virtual reality lab.

The desire among professors at medical schools to have 3-D models and other simulation technology goes back a long time. But it took a while for the technology to catch up to the vision. "To do graphics in real-time, three-dimensional ways takes a lot of computing power and takes some very sophisticated data,"[11] says Dr. Mark Whitehead, an anatomy professor at the University of California–San Diego medical school's Department of Surgery.

Anatomy class is but one place where VR technology is transforming a med school education. The operating room is also seeing more virtual patients. Future surgeons are getting experience in performing risk-free procedures with the help of virtual reality.

A Realistic Feel

The surgical training aspect of VR allows medical students to perform simulated surgeries on virtual patients. A Stanford University VR program, for example, uses CT scans to create a highly detailed simulated sinus surgery. A VR simulator developed at the University of Montreal, called SIM-K, helps students learn complicated knee-replacement procedures, complete with sensors that re-create the humming and vibrations of saws and drills.

Surgical Partners Miles Apart

One form of VR technology is connecting more experienced doctors with less experienced doctors during surgeries. This kind of arrangement is especially helpful for military surgeons, who often find themselves working in challenging conditions on injuries with which they have little experience. With the help of VR, a military surgeon near the action can transmit what he or she is seeing to a doctor on the other side of the world who can help the battlefield surgeon treat the patient. It is a form of telementoring, and it is not just for the military. Surgeons in rural America, developing nations, or anywhere with scant medical resources can benefit.

This telementoring system, developed at the University of Alabama–Birmingham, is called virtual interactive presence and augmented reality (VIPAR). The system includes a local station where surgery is taking place and a remote station manned by the experienced surgeon. The doctor at each station has a digital viewing piece that contains two cameras for stereoscopic image capture and a high-definition viewer showing a virtual field. As the local surgeon operates, the remote surgeon sees everything the local surgeon sees. The remote surgeon can warn about potential problems or explain how to get to hard-to-reach places. Before VIPAR, this kind of advice had to be delivered by phone or videoconferencing. But these had their limits. Now, with the ability of a remote veteran surgeon to see in real time what a counterpart is seeing and doing on the other side of the world, more people will be saved.

But instead of those tools, students and surgical residents use plastic tools and styluses that can manipulate the bone, muscle, and other tissue of the computer-generated knee joint on their monitors. "There's a realistic feeling about the instruments . . . when you move around the knee, if you hit the bone, you feel a firm sensation,"[12] says Felix Brassard, an orthopedic resident at Maisonneuve-Rosemont hospital in Montreal. He adds that this type of training should calm the nerves of surgeons when they finally operate on a living patient.

Even at centers where there are not yet sophisticated VR labs, medical students can get similar experience on mobile devices with surgical simulation apps. The Chicago-based tech company Level EX released its first app, Airway EX, in 2017. Video game developers took footage of real surgeries to create simulations of various procedures to treat blocked airways and other respiratory problems. The graphics and responses in the app, which is designed like a game with increasingly challenging levels, can be a little alarming, says Level EX chief executive officer (CEO) Sam Glassenberg. "It bleeds, it coughs, it reacts and it's running on a device you already own," Glassenberg says. "It's a totally reactive patient. . . . Right now, if you want to try out a new (surgical) device, they reserve a cadaver lab, or you use a mannequin in a room. But the beauty of this is you have it on a tablet or phone and it reacts, but it's not a live patient. It's perfectly safe. You can try things you never would."[13]

mannequin

in medical terms, a model of a human used to help teach others about how the body works

Lifesaving Steps Before Delicate Operations

But surgical VR programs are not just for med school students and residents still learning their craft. VR is helping established surgeons by allowing them to perform virtual operations or at least preview a specific patient's anatomy before the actual surgery. Dr. Gary Steinberg, a Stanford surgeon, says using VR to preview a delicate operation to treat a brain aneurysm was likely a lifesaving step for one patient because it revealed an artery attached to the top of the aneurysm. "You couldn't see it on conventional imaging," Steinberg says. "Had I not known about it, it could have been a real disaster. . . . Before, we didn't have the ability to reconstruct it in three dimensions; we'd have to do it in our minds. This way it's a three-dimensional rendering."[14]

aneurysm

a bulge in the wall of a blood vessel; an aneurysm that ruptures can be life-threatening

This type of 3-D imaging is especially helpful for surgeons working on complex and highly vulnerable organs, such as the brain. The medical VR company Surgical Theater developed a system in which imaging scans of a patient's brain are placed in a VR environment. A surgeon can slip on a pair of goggles and explore the brain of the patient to be operated on the next day. "We allow the pilot to fly through the scene of tomorrow's mission. And that's exactly what we're allowing a brain surgeon,"[15] says Surgical Theater CEO Moty Avisar.

Dr. Neil Martin, chair of the University of California–Los Angeles (UCLA) Department of Neurosurgery, and other neurosurgeons at UCLA have been using VR headsets for presurgery practice runs since 2014. For complex operations, in particular, knowing what to expect ahead of time can improve chances of success. Martin says:

> It's just amazing to see every little opening in the skull where a nerve goes through. I'm virtually inside the skull of the patient walking around, floating around. . . . On the image, I can see the carotid artery going through the margin of the tumor. . . . Rather than have that all of a sudden appear as I'm removing [the] tumor, I'll know exactly when I'm going to encounter it. That is a big improvement.[16]

Lucas Deines, whose surgeon used VR technology to preview the operation before actually removing a tumor from Deines's brain, later donned a VR headset at UCLA to see the tumor that had been removed. He summed up VR and medicine quite simply, saying, "It's like the convergence of gaming and lifesaving."[17]

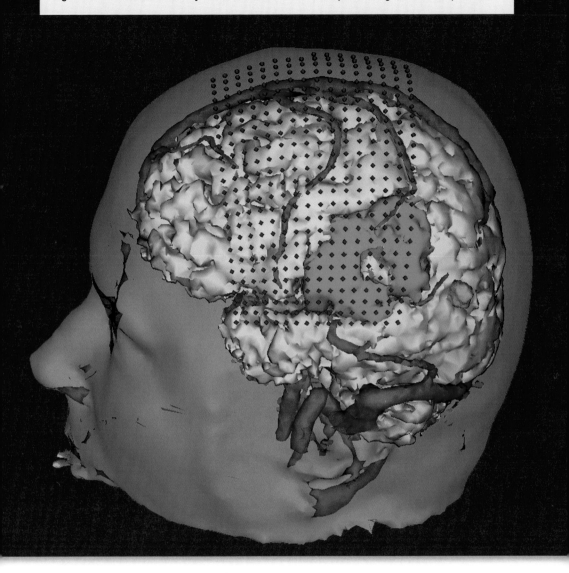

Three-dimensional imaging of the head helps doctors diagnose potential problems in their patients. Here, a 3-D head scan reveals a brain tumor (in green). Surgeons will study the image to determine the best way to remove the tumor before proceeding with a live operation.

A surgeon can also perform an operation while wearing a VR headset that is connected to the headsets worn by medical students. This allows a medical student to follow along, making the same moves as the surgeon. That was the case for Shafi Ahmed's groundbreaking surgery broadcast in VR. While he removed a cancerous tumor from a patient's colon, he explained what he was doing as twenty med students in a nearby classroom followed along, each with their own VR headsets. Surgeons are also

Med Students Experience Virtual Aging

Medical students in their twenties and thirties have only a secondhand understanding of what it means to grow old. They might work with older patients and have older family members, neighbors, and teachers. But now they can gain a better understanding of the challenges faced by older adults through a VR program called We Are Alfred. The program, developed by students at the University of Illinois–Chicago, helps med students experience life as an older adult with visual and hearing impairments as well as arthritis and other age-related physical challenges.

When students don the VR headset, their vision and hearing change. Suddenly, they see the way an older person with macular degeneration sees: Objects straight ahead appear to be blacked out. Hearing also becomes more difficult. Patients with poor vision and hearing are sometimes misdiagnosed as having dementia because of how they respond to a physician's questions and instructions. With simulations like We Are Alfred, the next generation of doctors may have greater insight and more empathy for their older patients.

wearing cameras that will capture their every move during surgery in order for video of those operations to be incorporated into VR surgical training simulations.

VR in Other Health Fields

Surgeons and medical school students are not the only health professionals who are benefiting from advances in virtual reality. Other physicians, paramedics, dentists, and nursing students are also getting valuable training with the help of VR technology.

Even experienced clinicians can benefit from ongoing education. A physician who has learned from textbooks and simply working with patients may still be challenged with certain complex medical conditions. Irritable bowel syndrome (IBS), a condition that affects the large intestine and causes abdominal pain and other uncomfortable symptoms, is one such problem. It has several potential causes, and people with IBS can experience symptoms differently. Salix, a pharmaceutical company, developed a VR platform that takes doctors through the various possible causes of IBS by leading them on a journey through the gastrointestinal tract. "As a gastroenterologist who treats conditions like IBS on a daily basis, I believe this virtual reality experience will move GI treatment forward by helping healthcare professionals better understand this complex condition,"[18] says Dr. Brooks Cash, chief of gastroenterology and director of the Gastroenterology Physiology Lab at the University of South Alabama Digestive Health Center.

Paramedics in training are using VR to learn lifesaving skills in non-life-threatening situations. But because VR environments can do such a good job re-creating the intensity of a real-world car accident, for example, paramedics are getting as close to the real thing as possible during their training. Emergency services workers in Palm Beach County, Florida, made VR a part of their

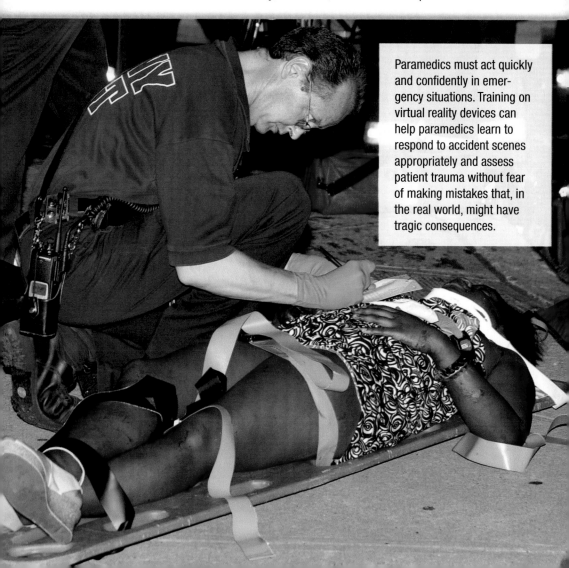

Paramedics must act quickly and confidently in emergency situations. Training on virtual reality devices can help paramedics learn to respond to accident scenes appropriately and assess patient trauma without fear of making mistakes that, in the real world, might have tragic consequences.

training, and the results have been steadier performance in actual emergencies. "They are much more calm in the field because they've seen it already," says fire department chief Cory Bessette. "It is so realistic, and it puts you in that scenario where there is a little bit of stress, where you're sweating a little bit, and you're trying to work through the scenario."[19]

Dental students are among the more recent converts to VR training. HapTEL, a haptic system that allows them to work on a virtual set of teeth and experience the vibrations and pressure of using a drill to remove decay, provides a comfort level that is essential when treating patients who are not always comfortable themselves in a dentist's chair. These haptic systems allow dental students to control the pressure, speed, and direction of drills and other instruments on the screen shared by a virtual patient's 3-D mouth and head.

Virtual patients are also helping nursing students. An instructor can create real-time simulations of a wide range of patient types for nursing students to diagnose and treat. John Miller, an online nursing instructor at Tacoma Community College in Washington State, says that giving his students virtual patients to treat and being able to control what the patient says and how the patient reacts is invaluable training. "Students can assess—and I can change—what happens to the patient,"[20] says Miller, adding that he can make a patient cough, talk, or have a medical emergency with just a click of a mouse.

While VR is playing an ever-increasing role in the training of health care professionals at all levels, it is still just one type of training tool. Training for students and experienced providers takes many forms. What makes VR stand out is the interactive nature of the experience. It is more involved than reading a book or listening to a lecture. Health experts see a long future for this technology, precisely because it is not a passive experience. "All of these activities are engaging, pulling the learner in, consuming their attention, allowing them to interact, and allowing them to take responsibility for their own education," says Robert Hasel, associate dean of simulation, immersion, and digital learning at Western University of Health Sciences. "This is similar to a person playing a video game; they are responsible for what they do in that environment; they take ownership to their education in that environment; and it is fun."[21]

CHAPTER 3

Studying and Treating the Brain

The brain is a fascinating machine, but doctors and researchers still have much to learn about how it functions and how best to deal with brain injuries or conditions that affect thinking and motor skills. Since VR is all about tricking the senses, it follows that this technology would find its way into the diagnosis and treatment of brain disorders and mental health conditions. A doctor studying the effects of brain surgery can have a patient wear a VR headset during surgery and then use the VR environment to stimulate certain senses of the patient to see how the brain responds. VR platforms help diagnose concussions and help patients recover from brain injuries, as well as cope with chronic conditions such as autism. And those are only a few examples of how VR is changing the fields of neurological and mental health. Brain health, perhaps more than any other field of medicine, may be the most directly influenced by advances in virtual reality.

neurological

relating to the structure, function, and diseases of the nervous system, including the brain

Patients undergoing brain surgery are sometimes kept awake during the operation because the surgeon needs to see whether the treatment is working or make sure that an incision is not affecting a part of the brain responsible for sight, hearing, speech, or movement. As an example, when removing a brain tumor that is near an area responsible for speech, the surgeon may ask the patient to answer a question to make sure that part of the brain is okay. At Angers University Hospital in France in 2016, surgeons performed a delicate operation to remove a tumor from a patient's brain. As was customary in this type of surgery, the patient was given a local anesthetic to prevent pain but was otherwise awake and alert.

What was unusual about this operation is that the patient was wearing a VR headset. Through the VR headset, a doctor working with the surgical team controlled what the patient saw and heard. In this case, controlling the patient's visual input was especially important. The tumor had affected at least one eye. So the VR environment the patient viewed through his goggles had lighted objects appear in his peripheral field of view. The doctors could see exactly how his brain and optic nerves were responding. Fortu-

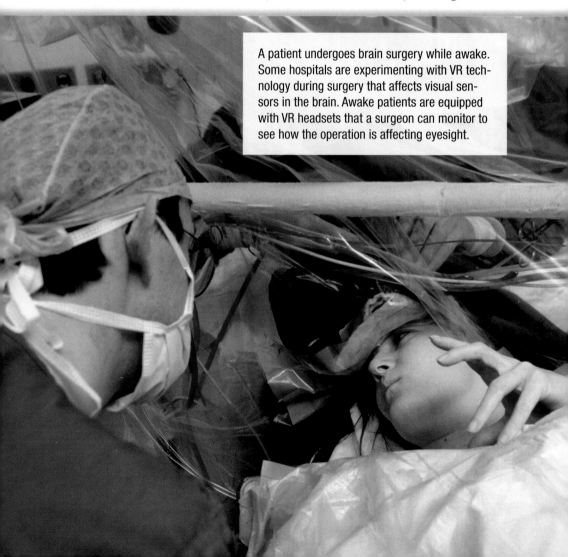

A patient undergoes brain surgery while awake. Some hospitals are experimenting with VR technology during surgery that affects visual sensors in the brain. Awake patients are equipped with VR headsets that a surgeon can monitor to see how the operation is affecting eyesight.

nately for that patient, the results were encouraging. Learning how a tumor or the surgery to remove one affects brain function is called brain mapping. The doctors at Angers University Hospital and elsewhere see VR as an especially helpful tool in brain mapping, and they plan to use it more for surgeries affecting sight and other senses. "By totally controlling what the patient sees and hears, we can put him in situations that allow us to do tests on certain connections that were not possible before,"[22] Angers University Hospital neurosurgeon Philippe Menei says.

brain mapping

the process of studying how a tumor or the surgery to remove one affects brain function

Advancing Understanding of Brain Function

Virtual reality has applications in brain research and medicine even beyond surgery. It has the capability to enhance understanding of this enormously complex organ. Neurons are special cells that carry signals within the brain and from the brain to other parts of the body. Scientists still have much to learn about how neurons, the basic units of the brain and nervous system, work. General Electric's Neuro VR is helping neurologists and neuropsychiatrists better visualize how neurons send and transmit information. "[It's] a very interactive and intuitive way of visualizing complex, multidimensional neuro imaging data," says Sandeep Gupta from GE Global Research. "A neurosurgeon could use tools like these to get a complete view of lesions and possible impact of surgery on brain networks and function."[23]

VR to Improve Brain Function

VR research may also lead to therapies that could help improve neuron activity associated with memory. Researchers at UCLA discovered that neurons in the hippocampus—the part of the brain associated with memory—behave differently in the real world compared to the virtual world. It is still not clear exactly why this occurs. The researchers learned about these different responses by analyzing the brain circuitry of rats in actual environments and virtual ones.

Mayank Mehta is a professor of physics, neurology, and neurobiology at UCLA and the lead author of several studies of VR and brain activity. He says that the more researchers understand the differences in neuron activity between real and virtual environments, the greater potential there is for treatment. Mehta explains that when the brain is learning or retrieving a memory, groups of neurons communicate using complex rhythm patterns, like the many instruments working together in an orchestra to play a symphony. Says Mehta:

> These complex rhythms are crucial for learning and memory, but we can't hear or feel these rhythms in our brain. They are hidden under the hood from us. The complex pattern they make defies human imagination. The neurons in this memory-making region talk to each other using two entirely different languages at the same time. One of those languages is based on rhythm; the other is based on intensity.[24]

Mehta adds that the language based on the intensity of the signals neurons exchange with each other becomes disrupted in virtual reality. A similar breakdown may be present in people with memory disorders. Mehta says that if researchers can identify what conditions in the virtual world can cause neuron dysfunction, that information may be useful in identifying causes of memory problems in the real world. Mehta says that if neuron rhythms and intensity in the hippocampus can be synchronized and improved with treatment, doctors may have a powerful weapon in the fight against dementia. VR research may be the key.

Diagnosing Brain Trouble

VR is already playing a role in diagnosing neurological problems or the extent of injuries that cause brain damage. Diagnosing such problems continues to present great challenges for doctors. But with VR, a person's decision-making and problem-solving skills can be tested in situations that mimic the real world instead of through the kinds of screenings patients typically do in a doctor's office, such as matching cards. The Wisconsin Card Sorting Test (WCST) is a common screening tool that psychologists use with

Empathy for Migraine Sufferers

Virtual reality games and movies are sometimes accused of inadvertently causing headaches. A VR program created by Excedrin, the company that makes pain-relief medications, actually simulates the symptoms of a real migraine headache—extreme sensitivity to light and sound, for example. The goal is to make people who do not experience migraines more empathetic to the millions who do. Non-migraine sufferers can put on an Excedrin headset and experience through augmented reality feelings of pressure in the head, sensitivity to light and sound, feelings of disorientation, and other migraine symptoms. Excedrin worked with migraine sufferers to capture their unique symptoms.

Diana Crandall, a reporter for the *New York Daily News*, tried the migraine simulator for an article in 2016. While she did not experience the searing pain and nausea that can accompany migraines, she did describe her experience as "nearly unbearable." She wrote, "I couldn't compose a text message, let alone scroll through a newsfeed. I sat helplessly trying to make a phone call." When she got up to walk, her VR headache made things even worse. "I staggered down my office hallway in a seemingly drunken stupor, grasping at walls to try and steady my steps. I could barely focus on putting one foot in front of the other, making talking while walking akin to a mission impossible."

Diana Crandall, "Daily Newser Tries Out Migraine Simulator So You Don't Have To," *New York Daily News*, April 9, 2016. www.nydailynews.com.

people who have had brain injuries or who have a form of mental illness or cognitive decline. In the test, patients are asked to match cards with different colored and numbered shapes. They can match cards by shapes, colors, or numbers. Only the person administering the test knows the kind of match being sought. If the patient is told that it is an incorrect match, he or she must figure out what the right match is without being told. In the VR version of this screening, a patient is trying to leave a building and must match certain doors based on color. A study of this VR platform found that it is just as effective at revealing problems with thinking skills and may even be more valid than the WCST because it puts the patient in a situation that is closer to the real world.

A different type of brain injury, a concussion, is also proving to be the kind of condition that strongly lends itself to VR diagnosis. A Boston-based company called SyncThink developed a concussion test that can be done in about a minute. Immediately after a football player or anyone who has suffered a potential concussion is hurt, a headset can be placed on the head and an eye-tracking test can begin. Certain types of equipment such as Oculus Rift or Gear VR will work. If the player cannot properly meet the eye-tracking test's requirements, the player and others can be alerted to the possibility of a concussion. This kind of scientific test can take the guesswork out of deciding whether a player can safely return to the action.

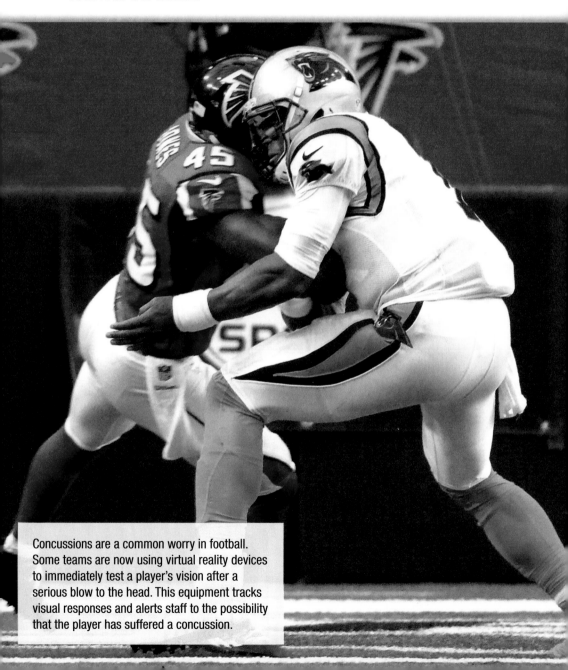

Concussions are a common worry in football. Some teams are now using virtual reality devices to immediately test a player's vision after a serious blow to the head. This equipment tracks visual responses and alerts staff to the possibility that the player has suffered a concussion.

VR technology is already being used to assess brain injuries by several professional sports teams and by doctors at the Walter Reed National Military Medical Center. "We can use this technology to help pinpoint the exact type of injury," says Sync-Think's chief technology officer, Daniel Beeler. "Head injury is complicated. A force to the head could involve brain damage. It could involve inner ear issues like balance. It could be other issues that produce similar symptoms. We want to provide objective technology to identify the specific issue at hand and improve outcomes."[25]

Understanding more about a brain injury is but one way VR is helping doctors and other health care providers diagnose and treat people with brain-related challenges. In some cases it is not an injury but a condition from childhood that can be managed better with some time spent in virtual reality.

Treating Autism

When a brain-related condition such as autism affects communication and other behaviors, VR can help with treatment there, too. Helping kids learn social cues and communication skills if they are on the autism spectrum is an especially robust field of VR in brain medicine. Autism (or autism spectrum disorder, as it is known clinically) is a mental condition that usually appears in childhood. People with autism, which can be mild or severe, sometimes have trouble communicating, understanding social cues, and maintaining friendships.

A VR-based program developed at the University of Texas–Dallas (UTD) measures brain waves while young people with autism go through simulated situations like being in a classroom or in a job interview. The program seems to improve activity in the areas of the brain responsible for social understanding. "Individuals with autism may become overwhelmed and anxious in social situations," says Dr. Nyaz Didehbani, a research clinician with the Center for Brain Health at UTD. "The virtual reality training platform creates a safe place for participants to practice social situations without the intense fear of consequence."[26]

Tandra Allen, who oversees virtual training programs at UTD, sees value in VR therapy for both children and adults, each of whom have specific challenges related to autism and their quality of life. She says:

> This research builds on past studies we conducted with adults on the autism spectrum and demonstrates that virtual reality may be a promising and motivating platform for both age groups. This was the first study to pair participants together with the goal of enhancing social learning. We observed relationships in life grow from virtual world conversations. We saw a lot of growth in their ability to initiate and maintain a conversation, interpret emotions and judge the quality of a friendship.[27]

Some of the virtual situations users were placed in include inviting someone to a party, meeting a peer for the first time, and dealing with a bully. Two clinicians led the people with autism through the programs. One clinician provided instructions and guidance, while the other played the part (through a virtual avatar) of the bully, new friend, or other character in the situation. Dr. Daniel Krawczyk, associate professor of cognitive neuroscience and cognitive psychology at UTD, says that VR therapy leads to improvements that can be harder to achieve in traditional classroom or clinical settings. "It's exciting that we can observe changes in diverse domains including emotion recognition, making social attribution, and executive functions related to reasoning through this life-like intervention," Krawczyk says. "These results demonstrate that core social skills can be enhanced using a virtual training method."[28]

cognitive

related to intellectual activity, such as learning, thinking, reasoning, and remembering

Improving Motor Skills and More

Studies have also shown that VR can help improve perception and motor skills in people with other neurological disorders, such as cerebral palsy. Cerebral palsy is a condition in which the part of the brain responsible for movement, balance, and muscle con-

Students Win Award for Virtual Reality Invention

At the Disrupt NY 2017 Hackathon, the first team to show off its product onstage was composed of three teenage girls. The New Jersey high school students had created re-VIVE, a virtual reality program designed to diagnose attention-deficit/hyperactivity disorder (ADHD). Making an accurate ADHD diagnosis is challenging, time consuming, and potentially quite expensive. The simulation tests a user's motor skills, reaction time, and sustained concentration. Tasks include touching objects when they turn a certain color, navigating through a maze, and standing still within a defined space. While not made with the goal of replacing mental health professionals trained to make this diagnosis, reVIVE could be a tool to help therapists get a better idea of a patient's strengths and weaknesses in those areas. What made the reVIVE team member's project especially impressive is that they accomplished it in twenty-four hours—the allotted time for teams to create their entries. The three teens won first prize (and collected a $5,000 check) for their effort.

trol is damaged or develops abnormally before or immediately after birth. A 2002 study of children with cerebral palsy playing VR learning games resulted in improved motor skills, learning ability, visual perception, and decision making. As part of the study, the children played virtual games including volleyball and soccer. To get virtual players to hit the volleyball over the net or block a shot into the soccer goal, the child had to move his or her arms in certain ways. These movements challenge and encourage visual perception and coordination. Another game, called Orbosity, featured a tranquil setting with a snowy mountain in the distance and brightly colored balls floating in the air. In this game, players earn points by virtually touching each ball. A hard touch causes the ball to burst into many colors. A too-soft touch causes the ball to turn into a bird that flies off the screen. The players keep track of their scores as they play, usually seeing improvement the longer they play. Researchers observed how the students performed and asked them afterward about their experiences. The fun and competitive nature of the games inspired the young cerebral palsy patients to play longer and try harder. And what was especially gratifying to the researchers was that the children liked having some control over their performance.

The feeling of having control over one's actions is especially important for people (no matter their age) who have a chronic disease or disability that prevents such control in daily life. Lead researcher Denise Reid, a professor of occupational therapy at the University of Toronto, explains: "This pilot study suggests that a virtual play environment provides children with an opportunity to interact with virtual play activities that are enjoyable and non-threatening. This opportunity allows for increased play engagement and an opportunity to exercise control over their actions. This overall experience enables the development of a sense of mastery or greater self-efficacy feelings."[29]

This is just one example of VR-based therapy that is being developed to improve life for people who have physical and, in some cases, mental challenges. Other researchers are working on similar therapies for people with Down syndrome, for example. Still other work is being done in an effort to control how the brain responds to stimuli.

Changing Brain Responses

Most brain and body responses are beyond a person's control. They happen automatically. When it is cold, a whole series of changes occur in the body. Shivering begins to generate heat. Circulation decreases in the extremities to ensure that the vital organs are well supplied and remain warm. But some responses to stimuli can be controlled, or at least shifted a little with some therapy. And now VR is a component of that work. For example, stress can trigger a desire to eat certain unhealthy foods. That can cause numerous health problems. Too much salt, for instance, can raise blood pressure.

A company called AppliedVR took on the challenge of training people's brains to respond more positively to stress. One approach, for instance, was to take users on a VR journey through a body harmed by unhealthy eating. "We wanted to help give them empathy for what was going on inside the body, where you can take them inside the body and give them perspective of what's happening inside their kidneys, inside their heart,"[30] says Applied-VR CEO Matthew Stoudt.

AppliedVR also makes VR systems to help spark memories in people who have Alzheimer's disease and other forms of dementia. A VR experience of certain sights and sounds can lead

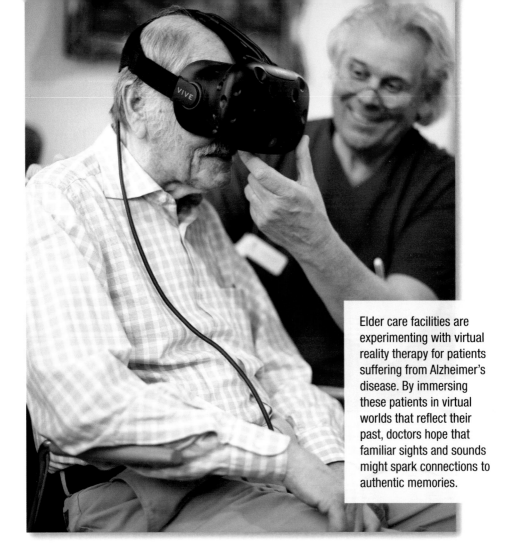

Elder care facilities are experimenting with virtual reality therapy for patients suffering from Alzheimer's disease. By immersing these patients in virtual worlds that reflect their past, doctors hope that familiar sights and sounds might spark connections to authentic memories.

a person to recall personal memories and share them with loved ones. This concept follows an established therapy for dementia patients in which familiar songs and scrapbooks are used to help spark memory retrieval.

With all the brain research employing VR-based technology going on around the world, experts predict remarkable changes in the diagnosis and treatment of neurological conditions in the years ahead. "It's estimated that our knowledge [of the brain] is about 50 years behind that of every other organ in our body," says Cory Strassburger, cofounder of Kite & Lightning, a VR content studio. But he believes that is going to change. "The beauty is this big mystery inside our brain is just beginning to unfold and I think VR will play an important role on both the scientific and educational sides."[31]

CHAPTER 4

Easing Pain and Anxiety

Since its earliest days as an entertainment medium, one of the most widely used VR environments has been a virtual roller coaster. There are dozens of twisting, turning, stomach-churning VR rides you can take on home VR systems, as well as at huge theme parks such as SeaWorld Orlando and Six Flags New England. A VR roller coaster offers all the sensations of a real roller coaster, but a person can get off at any time—a big advantage, some might say, for people who are afraid of these increasingly fast and furious rides. That same idea of putting people in virtual environments that they find scary or upsetting is at the heart of therapies that use VR to treat phobias, anxiety, addictions, PTSD, and other mental health issues. VR is also being used to help patients cope with physical health challenges, such as pain, and the monotony that accompanies long hospital stays. Sometimes an escape to a virtual world is the best medicine.

> **debilitating**
>
> impaired strength and vitality, often caused by an illness or disorder

Phobia Therapy

Fear of flying is a real and debilitating condition that afflicts more than 6 percent of the US population (though some estimates place the figure much higher). Treatment for this condition usually involves counseling to help people better understand and cope with their fear. But hypnosis, medications, and other methods have also been used, with mixed results. Clinics around the world are now using virtual reality to treat this phobia, and it is showing remarkable success.

In a virtual reality environment, a patient sits in a standard commercial airline seat nervously waiting for his or her flight to take off. The patient's feet will not actually leave the earth, but he or she will see, hear, and even feel all the sensations of a big jet taking off, soaring through the clouds, and landing safely. Clinics around the world take patients through these simulated flights on a regular basis. The patients wear VR headsets to re-create real-life flights, while a therapist controls the action, offers calming advice, and repeats scary situations in a controlled environment until the patient can better cope with the fear of flying. If flying in bad weather is the problem, those conditions can also be simulated in a way that will help ease fear and anxiety. "This could be a real revolution in clinical care,"[32] says Albert "Skip" Rizzo, director of Medical Virtual Reality at the University of Southern California's Institute for Creative Technologies.

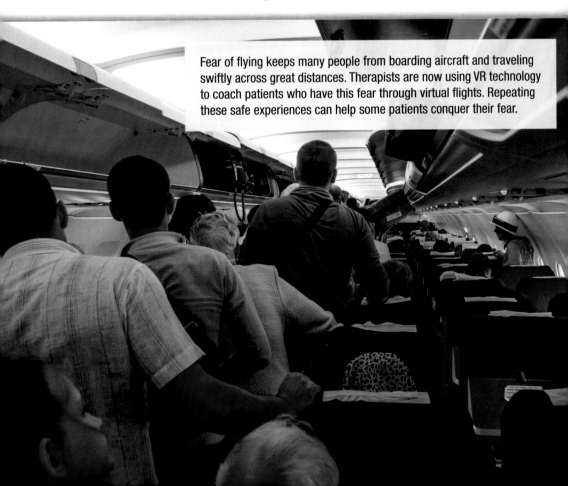

Fear of flying keeps many people from boarding aircraft and traveling swiftly across great distances. Therapists are now using VR technology to coach patients who have this fear through virtual flights. Repeating these safe experiences can help some patients conquer their fear.

Fear of flying is only one such phobia being treated with VR. Psychiatrists are finding that with VR, a patient can be exposed to an environment normally associated with a deep-seated fear, and one that normally triggers great anxiety. Fear of confined spaces, fear of heights, fear of public speaking, and other phobias all have VR-based treatments. These treatments are called exposure therapy, and they are a rapidly growing trend in psychology. Colorado psychologist Dawn Jewell used VR to treat a patient who had an awful car crash and had a paralyzing fear of returning to the intersection where the crash occurred. With Limbix, a company that provides exposure therapy programs for Google's Daydream View headset, Jewell could join the patient on a virtual trip through that intersection. "It provides exposure in a way that patients feel safe," Jewell says. "We can go to a location together, and the patient can tell me what they're feeling and what they're thinking."[33]

Treatment for Emotional Trauma

The reason VR is so effective in treating anxiety is that it can create "emotionally evocative experiences," says Rizzo. His work

Meditation Made Easier with Virtual Reality

Meditation is commonly used to help reduce stress in people who are experiencing emotional and physical challenges. And virtual reality has a role to play in meditation. It can be used to teach meditation techniques. It can also provide a more in-depth sensory experience as a person relaxes into a meditative state.

One advantage of using VR for meditation is that the user can be completely immersed in a visual and auditory environment specifically designed to bring on calm and mindfulness. That environment might be a tropical island, a Japanese temple, or some other peaceful setting. Rather than seeing laundry waiting to be folded or a messy desk covered with unfinished homework, users immerse themselves in the simulated environment.

One VR game, called *DEEP*, helps users learn deep-breathing exercises while calming the mind. The VR environment is a relaxing undersea world. For this game, in addition to the usual VR headset, users wear a sensor on a strap around the chest that measures diaphragm expansion to check breathing. Only through proper deep breathing and sinking into a further meditative state can users move from one level of the game to another.

in developing simulations for PTSD patients, especially military veterans, earned him the American Psychological Association's 2010 Award for Outstanding Contributions to the Treatment of Trauma. "With PTSD and phobias, you have people who are very primed to react to stimuli that remind them of what they went through or what they fear," Rizzo says. "It has to do with the user's history and the emotional reactivity to the stimuli."[34]

> **evocative**
>
> bringing strong feelings, memories, or images to mind

He explains that a person who has never been in a combat situation will have a much different experience in a VR wartime simulation than a veteran who has served on the front lines. He recalls an early 1990s Vietnam War simulation created by a colleague, Barbara Rothbaum, with primitive graphics and sound effects. Those things did not matter, however. "When you asked the people who had served in Vietnam what they thought of the experience, they talked about seeing the Viet Cong hiding in the jungle, tracer fire, seeing a water buffalo by the river," Rizzo says. "Except none of those things were in the simulation. They brought those memories to the experience."[35]

These days VR can re-create in great detail the kinds of traumatic experiences that give vets nightmares and other coping challenges. In a safe, controlled environment, the veterans can be coached to deal with these thoughts and images in a healthy way as they are reliving traumatic incidents. And each VR experience can be tailored to the particular user. The vet dons a headset with a prescribed "world," such as a desert highway or a marketplace. A clinician working the controls of the simulation talks with the user while he or she recounts the details of an attack or other event. The clinician may ask if the episode happened at night. If so, the VR environment can be adjusted to seem like night. Was the user driving a Humvee or in the front passenger seat? Was there debris along the road? Was it loud? Were there helicopters overhead? And so on. With every answer, the clinician adjusts the environment so it resembles as closely as possible the situation triggering the frightening flashbacks. Some of the more sophisticated systems have technology that causes the user's seat to rumble during an explosion in the simulation. There are even systems that can pipe in dozens of smells, such as diesel fuel and burning rubber tires. And, while the look of a VR environment is important, the sound detail and quality are just as important in a PTSD simulation. Rizzo says that there seem to be fewer and fewer skeptics about how effective VR can be at provoking emotional responses. Usually, it does not take long, even using a simple VR headset and program, to become a believer. "The human brain has an amazing ability to suspend disbelief," says Rizzo. "We cry at movies after all."[36]

limbic system
the parts of the brain that control long-term memory, emotion, behavior, and sense of smell

Virtual reality can allow someone to really imagine being in another place. It does this by simulating the sights, sounds, and smells that trigger strong responses in the brain's limbic system. This includes the parts of the brain most responsible for emotion (the amygdala) and memory (the hippocampus). "Your frontal lobe says you're not on top of that tall building, or in a room full of spiders, or in that airplane, but your limbic system kind of takes over,"[37] Rizzo says.

VR solutions work even for less debilitating fears. A study of schoolchildren in California looked at whether virtual reality could help allay the anxiety they felt about getting their seasonal flu shots. In a group of 244 kids, about half were fitted with VR goggles and watched relaxing ocean scenes. Not surprisingly, the children in the VR group reported less fear and pain compared to those who had no VR distraction.

Prescription for Pain

Distraction is actually one of VR's most effective features. Hospital patients often face more than anxiety during and after their procedures. Physical pain from a surgical incision or from an injury, such as a burn or fracture, may seem too real to be treated with any kind of virtual reality. In fact, VR is proving to be an effective distraction from pain. A surgeon in Mexico, for example, fits some patients with a VR headset prior to an operation and sends them on journeys to Peru's mysterious Machu Picchu and other faraway destinations. Depending on the procedure, a patient may be given just a local anesthetic, rather than the heavy sedatives and painkillers that are typically given before and after surgery. Dr. Jose Luis Mosso Vazquez sees this approach as having two big benefits: reducing the cost of medications and reducing the risk of side effects some patients have after being heavily medicated. Mosso says the idea for VR as a pain distraction during surgery came from a VR Spider-Man game his son received in 2004. "His Mom called him to go to dinner and he didn't hear her, nothing," Mosso says. "I thought, what if I use this on a patient?"[38]

VR games as distractions from pain take many forms. In the game *Bear Blast*, a user wearing a VR headset turns from side to side to throw colorful balls at bears encountered in this virtual environment. Brennan Spiegel directs health services research at Cedars-Sinai Medical Center in California. He notes that research found that patients who spend twenty minutes with *Bear Blast*

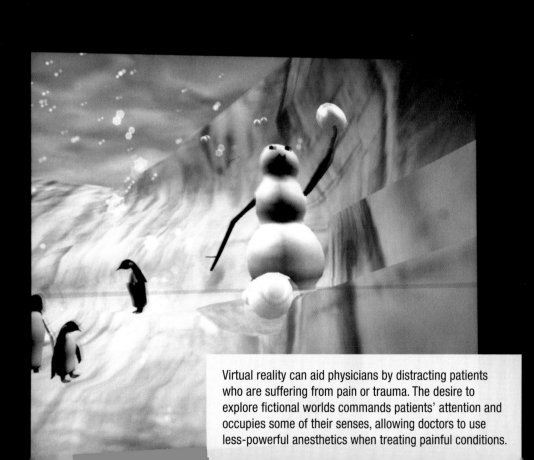

Virtual reality can aid physicians by distracting patients who are suffering from pain or trauma. The desire to explore fictional worlds commands patients' attention and occupies some of their senses, allowing doctors to use less-powerful anesthetics when treating painful conditions.

reported an average of a 24 percent reduction in pain. Before using VR, patients had an average pain score of roughly 5.5 on a scale of 0 to 10, but after VR therapy it averaged 4.0. "That's a pretty dramatic reduction for an acute pain," Spiegel says. "It's not too different from what we see from giving narcotics."[39]

Spiegel and others who have seen VR's impact on patient pain are encouraged that virtual reality may provide a nonaddictive, safe alternative to opioid painkillers, which are blamed for an epidemic of addiction, overdose, and other health problems. VR can be an effective distraction that can divert the brain's attention away from pain. A 2016 study in Tennessee found that just a five-minute experience in a VR game called *Cool!* resulted in an average reduction in temporary pain of 33 percent. *Cool!* takes players through a winter wonderland environment in which they can rack up points by hitting targets with snowballs. Study participants had lower back pain, hip pain, and other causes of chronic pain. The users had high praise for the technology and for the distraction from their pain. The researchers noted that the average age of study participants was fifty, which suggests that a video game approach to VR pain therapy can be effective among people who may be older than the traditional video game user.

VR games help distract from pain because focusing on the action in a game requires a considerable amount of attention. That means the brain has less attention to focus on the pain. "The

Treating Addiction

Medical specialists are experimenting with virtual reality as part of addiction treatment. At the University of Houston, heroin addicts are placed in a virtual setting that resembles a kitchen where they might be cooking up a batch of the drug or a party where people are huddled in a bathroom snorting heroin. This VR program is based on the idea that treating an addict in a lifelike setting works better than treatment in a medical clinic or office. In a virtual setting, addicts encounter realistic (but not real) triggers for their drug cravings, including drugs, drug paraphernalia, and other users. A therapist can monitor those heightened cravings and offer advice and coping strategies in the moment. This process can help addicts learn and put to use the coping skills they will need when they encounter these same triggers in the real world.

experience of pain is two-fold: physical stimuli or what's actually causing the pain and perception and processing," Rizzo says. "The perception of pain is dependent on what has our attention."[40] He adds, however, that while distraction is often effective in treating acute pain, such as injury recovery, VR plays a different role in treating chronic pain. Someone who lives with knee or back pain from arthritis or some other chronic condition needs techniques to cope with the discomfort. Relaxation exercises can help a person de-stress and find a distraction that does not require VR goggles. Rizzo explains:

> With chronic pain, you can't walk around with a headset all the time. Instead, you use a VR environment to teach strategies we know work in the real world. It's called meditation or mindfulness. Some people don't take the time because they don't think it will work. But with VR, you can be in an idyllic setting, like a mountaintop or beach, and have a soft voice doing guided imagery. It's more of a teaching situation.[41]

Virtual Reality Recovery

After an operation or during a treatment that requires a prolonged hospital stay, the problem is often boredom more than physical discomfort. Hospitals such as Cedars-Sinai in Los Angeles are providing patients with VR equipment to take them to far-off places, art museums, and elsewhere. This helps reduce the stress of a long hospital stay and provides a distraction from the discomfort the patient is enduring. Other VR programs are helping teen chemotherapy patients focus on games, rather than their treatment. At C.S. Mott Children's Hospital in Michigan, these programs are very popular because they allow a young patient to feel as though he or she is able to get out of the hospital—at least for a while. VR experiences include exploration of a rain forest, running down the tunnel before a football game at Michigan Stadium, and riding a roller coaster. The hospital also provides its young patients with augmented reality simulations that bring books to life and allow them to chase Pokémon with the AR game *Pokémon GO*.

Long-term hospital patients who may be missing out on a little brother's birthday party or a granddaughter's recital are also getting some VR assistance. A Dutch company is making that separation a little easier by combining VR and smartphone technologies to allow immersive contact between patients and their homes, schools, or other locations. VisitU uses a 360-degree camera at a remote location that transmits images back to the person wearing a VR headset in the hospital. A young patient can virtually walk around the room or other location containing the camera, creating the feeling of actually being present.

Previews for Patients

Sentiments such as boredom and feeling left out of important moments at home are common among hospitalized patients. Fear is another common emotion. Patients awaiting surgery, for instance, might fear the operation, the recovery, and the prospect of pain.

Through a virtual reality education experience, surgical patients get a complete run-through of their upcoming procedures before they even check into the hospital. This has become a popular feature at Tufts Medical Center in Boston. "The idea is to make sure patients are familiar with what they're about to undergo," says Carey Kimmelstiel, director of the hospital's Interventional Cardiology Center. "It doesn't have to be a scary process."[42]

Wearing VR goggles, a patient gets a 360-degree view of the surgical area and the hospital staff. The VR program takes viewers through the preprocedural consent process; introduces them to the doctors, nurses, and other health care providers; and explains the medical equipment involved in the procedure. The hope is that with this kind of exposure to the surgical experience in a calm setting, patients will be more relaxed. This should be especially helpful for patients who will not be under anesthesia, so they will be aware of their environment during the procedure. "It's a work in progress, but the technology is truly astounding," Kimmelstiel says. "When you're using it, you're not limited to a screenshot. You can really get a feel for the space. We'll be able to tell hesitant patients, 'Go home at your leisure, take a look at this, and think about questions you might not have thought to ask earlier.'"[43]

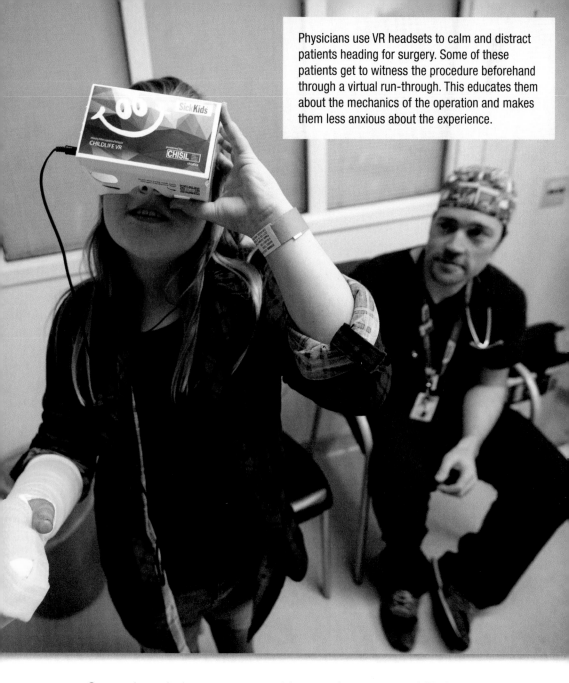

Physicians use VR headsets to calm and distract patients heading for surgery. Some of these patients get to witness the procedure beforehand through a virtual run-through. This educates them about the mechanics of the operation and makes them less anxious about the experience.

Some hospitals are even taking patients on a VR journey through the parts of their body that will undergo surgery. These patients go through the same VR simulation that a surgeon might do prior to surgery. Patient Sandi Rodoni took a VR tour of the blood vessels in her brain before a 2017 surgery at Stanford to repair a brain aneurysm. It was the same virtual journey taken by her surgeon, who noted clearly where a clip would be implanted to prevent the aneurysm from rupturing. It would be Rodoni's third such surgery. "Because I had been through this before, I thought I knew it all until I saw this," she said as she watched the images on her VR goggles. "I felt better knowing it was so clear to the doctor."[44]

Easing anxiety and distracting patients from pain in the real world are two major benefits provided by simulated virtual reality environments. Researchers continue to learn more about how to make virtual reality even more effective at helping people through emotional and physical traumas. Virtual reality will not replace traditional patient care. But by working side by side, VR specialists and health care providers can make a positive difference in the lives of suffering people around the world.

CHAPTER 5

Easing the Challenges of Recovery

The real-world challenges of recovering from a stroke, amputation, or brain injury can be overwhelming. Rehabilitation can be tedious, time consuming, and painful. While there are many established tools and techniques for helping with the rehabilitation process, virtual reality is gaining support as a new and valuable tool. When it comes to creating virtual worlds, just about anything is possible. Through the use of virtual reality, amputees are finding relief from phantom limb pain, and stroke patients and people who have experienced traumatic brain injuries are learning to walk and move more easily in the real world.

Regaining Movement After a Stroke

Strokes are serious and often deadly. A stroke occurs when a blood vessel that carries oxygen and nutrients to the brain is blocked by a clot or ruptures. When that happens, blood and oxygen stop flowing to the brain. This causes brain cells to die. Depending on the part of the brain affected by the stroke, the individual might lose control over one or both sides of the body, the ability to speak, and some thinking skills. Patients who survive a stroke sometimes need to relearn the use of their arms or legs. Intensive physical therapy, which involves repetitive actions over what can be a lengthy period of time, is often needed. Virtual reality can relieve the pain, frustration, and monotony of that process.

Some forms of stroke rehab involve mirror therapy. A person looks into a full-length mirror while standing on one foot or making various arm motions. This is a simple but common exercise in physical therapy to help patients improve their balance and coordination. Seeing themselves helps patients retain their balance and check to see if the actions are correct. But relearning to stand, walk, and maintain balance can take a long, frustrating time for stroke survivors. Seeing themselves struggle in a mirror can be discouraging for some people.

A company called GestureTek is offering a twist on this rehab exercise. It has designed a virtual reality version of mirror therapy. Instead of the patient sitting or standing in front of a mirror, the patient enters a virtual environment in which, for example, arm exercises might include virtual juggling in a circus setting, stopping shots as a soccer goalie, keeping balloons from hitting the

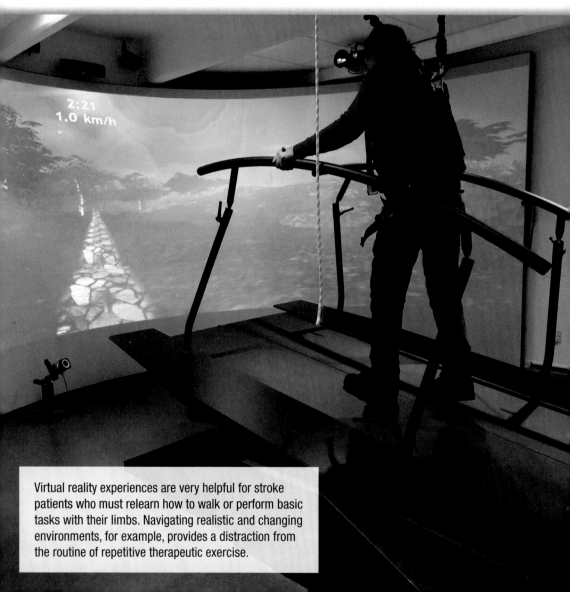

2:21
1.0 km/h

Virtual reality experiences are very helpful for stroke patients who must relearn how to walk or perform basic tasks with their limbs. Navigating realistic and changing environments, for example, provides a distraction from the routine of repetitive therapeutic exercise.

ground, and even playing a musical instrument. The patient is not really juggling or doing those other activities. And, in all likelihood, the patient's arms probably are not even moving very much at first. But in this therapy program, small movements in the real world translate to larger movements in the virtual world. The patient feels as though he or she is making real progress, which builds confidence and the desire to continue the exercises until the brain and body actually do make progress. "With VR, a little movement of the arm that's impaired creates a big movement (on the screen)," Albert "Skip" Rizzo says. "The focus is on the movement, not the limitation. They see things in feedback in the game, they'd never see in real life."[45] Eventually, those movements get bigger and more precise in the real world, too.

What is more, with this virtual version of mirror therapy, the tedious rehab process becomes almost fun. This is another way to keep people engaged in their therapy. Repetition is critical to successful physical therapy. Rizzo likens rehab to learning a musical instrument. "You have to work at it," he says. "You have to practice to get better. VR can give people feedback that will help keep them motivated."[46] If doing physical therapy in a virtual setting means a patient will do twenty more repetitions of an exercise or will work at the exercises for sixty minutes rather than thirty, this is a good outcome.

VR exercises and interactive games are not a replacement for conventional physical therapy. Rather, they nicely complement more traditional methods. This was the finding of a 2015 review of thirty-seven studies involving stroke rehab that included VR as part of the therapy. VR-based exercises at times led to greater improvements in limb function than standard therapy. But, the researchers emphasize, other traditional forms of therapy also benefited stroke patients.

Tracking Progress

Virtual reality offers other benefits to people recovering from stroke and other conditions that affect the brain. Some VR programs enable therapists to accurately track improvement in a patient's flexibility and strength over time. For example, changes in flexibility can be measured with each VR therapy session for a patient who is struggling to regain the use of an arm. As the arm gradually improves, the patient's VR file will display the degree of flexibility recorded in each session. Like swimmers who see their times improving the more they train, patients can see improvement by looking at the actual measurements of their increasing flexibility. This can be strong motivation to continue.

Eran Orr, founder of the Israel-based VRPhysio, says gathering data during the simulations also helps the therapists. They learn a patient's pain point or how far a patient has come with strength and flexibility and coordination training since the beginning of therapy. "We get four gigabytes of data from a session," Orr says. "We get data on how you are performing, and we can pass that on to the doctor or the insurance company."[47] That information can help determine whether an employee can safely return to work or whether an athlete is ready to play again. Orr and others in his field envision a time when VR-based rehab is just a standard part of injury recovery. VR headsets may become as standard as any other piece of therapeutic equipment.

Full-Bodied VR Technology

VR systems have demonstrated benefits for people who are undergoing rehabilitation for conditions other than stroke. This includes spinal cord injuries that lead to paralysis. A spinal cord injury involves damage to any part of the spinal cord or the nerves at the end of the spinal canal that affect sensation and body function in the lower half of the body. With many spinal cord injuries, the damage does not include a complete tear of the nerve bundles necessary for movement and sensation in the lower body. Instead, the bundle may have been partly crushed, leaving some nerves destroyed and others only injured.

exoskeleton

an external skeleton or shell that supports an animal's body; human-made exoskeletons can be used to help patients learn to walk after injuries

There are now VR systems that use a brain-controlled exoskeleton (sort of like Iron Man's suit) to help people who are paralyzed regain sensation and improve motor control. Patients begin this therapy by entering a virtual world, where they imagine themselves walking. These thoughts are transmit-

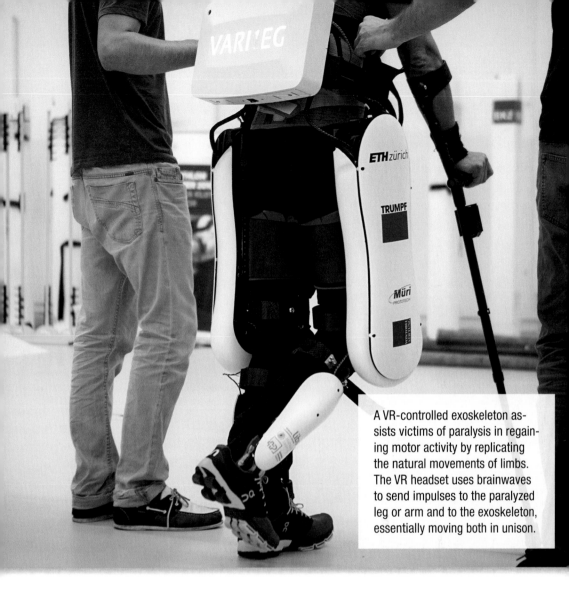

A VR-controlled exoskeleton assists victims of paralysis in regaining motor activity by replicating the natural movements of limbs. The VR headset uses brainwaves to send impulses to the paralyzed leg or arm and to the exoskeleton, essentially moving both in unison.

ted to an avatar, which moves as the person would move if he or she were able. Brain signals are recorded. The device, called the Brain-Machine Interface, converts those recordings into commands for the avatars. The machine even sends a mild vibration through the arms of the user with each step to reinforce the sensation of walking on a hard surface. After more of this training, the patient is helped into an exoskeleton programmed to follow those same thought commands.

In one British study, several people who were completely paralyzed were upgraded to partially paralyzed by the end of the year-long therapy using the exoskeleton and VR therapy. By working the limbs with an exoskeleton, injured nerves may be able to grow

Surfing in the Virtual World

Thirty-seven-year-old Danny Kurtzman has long wished he could surf. But Kurtzman, a Newport Beach, California, native who still calls the area home, has muscular dystrophy, a lifelong disease that causes a loss of muscle mass and weakness over time. Kurtzman uses a wheelchair; he cannot stand or walk. Despite his condition, Kurtzman got to experience the thrill of surfing in 2015. He did this through a virtual reality simulation developed by a company called Specular Theory. For the first time in his life, Kurtzman felt the excitement of standing on his board and surfing the waves. It did not matter that it was a virtual reality simulation. "It gave me that awesome feeling—that butterfly happiness feeling," Kurtzman says. "It allowed me to experience something I thought I never could experience."

Quoted in Lindsey Hoshaw, "Affordable Virtual Reality Opens New Worlds for People with Disabilities," NPR, October 22, 2015. www.npr.org.

healthy again, explains Brazilian neuroscientist Miguel Nicolelis. He is doing similar research at Duke University in North Carolina. He is encouraged that therapy that allows a patient's thoughts to control equipment such as the exoskeleton could represent a great leap forward for people who are paralyzed. The early results of Nicolelis's work are promising, with several patients regaining sensation and some movement in their legs. "I am very hopeful that we will be able to share these details with spinal rehab centers around the world," Nicolelis says. "If it works with spinal cord injuries, it may work with other injuries such as stroke."[48]

Distraction from the Pain of Walking

Virtual reality can help get patients walking more even when the problem has to do with their circulation and not their nerves or muscles. A condition called peripheral artery disease (PAD) can cause people a lot of pain when they walk. PAD means that one or more arteries that deliver oxygen-rich blood to the legs (or less frequently the arms or trunk) have become narrowed. This is often the result of cholesterol plaque building up along the walls of the arteries. Too much plaque means there is less room for blood to flow. And when a person's muscles get too little oxygen from blood, they get sore when they are being used. People with serious cases of PAD can develop leg pain after walking for only a few minutes.

A Dutch company called Beyond Care created a VR program to help distract PAD patients from their leg pain. Called Motivational Walk VR, it is designed to help distract PAD sufferers while they walk on a treadmill. The goal is to help people with PAD push past their pain limits. The more individuals with PAD can exercise, the longer they will be able to go before leg pain sets in. In the Motivational Walk VR environment, the therapist plants a virtual flag as the goal for the patient. Then the patient, wearing a headset, takes a walk down a pleasant path or trail toward that flag in the distance. The therapist can make each walk a little longer, and the VR environment can distract patients from the pain just enough so they do not mind taking a longer stroll.

> **phantom pain**
>
> an illusion of something that seems real but is not

Fighting Phantom Limb Pain

Virtual reality's unique ability to manipulate the senses is being applied to another area of injury and illness recovery. Individuals who have undergone amputation—of an arm or leg, a hand or foot, or even fingers or toes—often experience what is known as phantom limb pain. This is the sensation of pain in a part of the body that is no longer there. Medical researchers believe this results from the brain adjusting to having nerves severed during the amputation. "The tactile representation of different body parts are arranged in the brain in a sort of map," says Bo Geng, a medical VR developer and faculty member at Aalborg University in Denmark. "If the brain no longer receives feedback from an area, it tries to reprogram its signal reception map. That is the most common conception of how phantom limb pain occurs."[49]

> **tactile**
>
> relating to the sense of touch

When a person loses a limb and the nerves that went with it, other nerves in the body can send signals to the brain that make the brain feel that the missing limb is tightening and clenching.

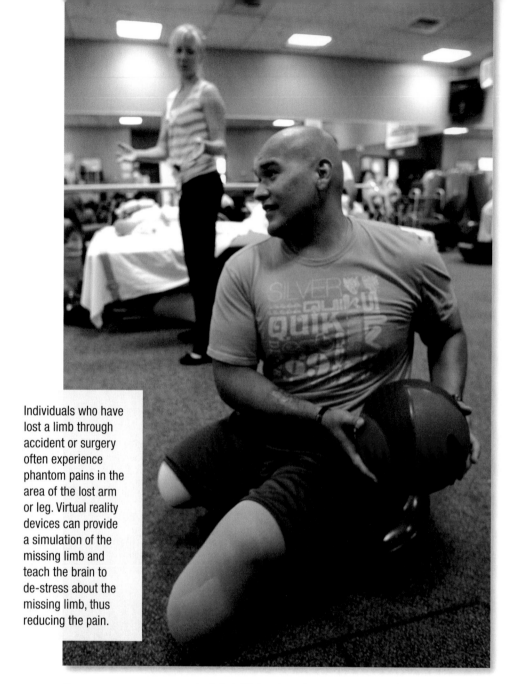

Individuals who have lost a limb through accident or surgery often experience phantom pains in the area of the lost arm or leg. Virtual reality devices can provide a simulation of the missing limb and teach the brain to de-stress about the missing limb, thus reducing the pain.

It can seem very painful. VR technology can provide individuals with a virtual limb and guide them through sessions where they learn to relax their virtual muscles and ease the discomfort being signaled by the brain's pain receptors.

Geng is using VR to give a traditional approach to treating phantom limb pain a fascinating twist. Mirror therapy, often used for people who have had a stroke, is also commonly used for treating amputees. It involves seating an amputee in front of a mirror. If that amputee is missing a left arm, the reflected image in the mirror is of a person with a working left arm and a missing right arm. As the person moves the right arm, it will appear in the reflection as though the left arm is the one that is moving. These movements can sometimes trick the brain into thinking it is still in contact with the missing left arm. Because the brain no longer feels the stress triggered by the loss of sensation from the missing limb's nerves, phantom limb pain subsides.

In a VR setting, that same amputee can put on the goggles and a glove on the remaining hand. Small electrodes are placed on the stump of the amputated limb, also known as the residual limb. During the VR simulation, the electrodes will administer small electrical charges to the residual limb, with the goal of re-creating some sensation in that limb. This provides the brain with further evidence that the missing limb is still there. When that sensation is paired with seeing the simulated limb move,

A VR Glove Improves Hand Function

Fine motor control in the fingers is essential for buttoning buttons, writing, texting, and myriad other tasks. Stroke, cerebral palsy, brain injury, and various developmental disabilities can make it hard to get fingers and thumbs working together. But VR has some solutions. Therapeutic gloves, with no goggles or headsets required, can help improve hand function.

Flint Rehab's MusicGlove, for example, takes a cue from the classic video game *Guitar Hero*. Each finger on the glove is fitted with a sensor. While wearing the glove, the user plugs it into a computer and presses play. Colorful circles appear at the top of the screen and then fall into matching circles at the bottom of the screen. Each color corresponds to a different note and to a different fingertip sensor. Each finger sensor has a color to match the colors of the circles on the screen. The order of the circles' appearance depends on the notes in the song that is playing. Once the moving circles match up, the user presses the matching colored fingertip sensor and thumb together.

Research shows that hand function can start to improve within two weeks of starting MusicGlove therapy. The movements help rewire the brain to compensate for injured nerves.

the brain thinks a functioning limb is still there, and thus no pain is felt. Geng says:

> The mirror therapy has some limitations because you have to physically sit down in front of a mirror, do the same movement in a confined space with both hands at the same time and keep your eyes on the mirror. The illusion can be easily broken. With virtual reality, there is a much better chance of creating a convincing alternative reality. Even though a person who has had a hand amputated can no longer see it, in many cases he or she can still feel it. This sensory conflict may be interpreted by the brain as pain. With this new method we try to overcome that conflict by providing an artificial visual and tactile feedback and in that way suppress the pain.[50]

Virtual Reality Fosters Hope

Advances in virtual reality are already giving hope to people who have had strokes and brain injuries or who suffer from an array of other health problems. But this technology is not yet widely available. Much of it is still experimental or in early stages of testing. Commercially available VR headsets and goggles—such as the Oculus Rift, HTC Vive, and Samsung Gear VR—can do many things in entertainment and education. But much more work is needed before these technologies have widespread applications in health and medicine.

The future of VR in medical science will depend on the changing needs of patients and doctors as well as on the companies and individuals who are on the cutting edge of this technology. Great innovations will emerge when designers and doctors can provide a useful VR experience for the people who need the help. Inventors at Samsung, for example, have developed a VR system that helps visually impaired people see more clearly. And research is under way at medical schools and high-tech incubators around the world on how to use VR to diagnose unusual diseases and make complex surgeries safer and accessible to people who do not live near well-equipped hospitals. "We're not going to virtualize everything," Rizzo says. But "with good theory and science in VR, we'll see people heal, get stronger, perform better, and live better in the real world."[51]

SOURCE NOTES

Introduction: Virtual Reality Transforms Medicine

1. Quoted in Cara McGoogan and Madhumita Murgia, "Watch the World's First Surgery Streamed in Virtual Reality Live from London," *Telegraph* (London), April 14, 2016. www.telegraph .co.uk.
2. Quoted in Jennifer Jolly, "Doctors Are Saving Lives with VR," *USA Today*, July 28, 2017. www.usatoday.com.

Chapter 1: A History of Illusion

3. Ivan E. Sutherland, "The Ultimate Display," Proceedings of IFIP Congress, 1965. http://worrydream.com/refs/Sutherland %20-%20The%20Ultimate%20Display.pdf.
4. Quoted in CBS News, "From Virtual Reality to Medical Reality," June 6, 2000. www.cbsnews.com.
5. Quoted in Sveta McShane, "How to Train Thousands of Surgeons at the Same Time in Virtual Reality," Singularity Hub, October 14, 2016. https://singularityhub.com.
6. Quoted in Barry Levine, "Forceps? Scalpel? Google Glass?," VentureBeat, March 12, 2014. https://venturebeat.com.

Chapter 2: Training Tool

7. Quoted in Rodney Tanaka, "Western U Pilot Tests Anatomage Navigator," press release, Western University of Health Sciences, April 27, 2016. www.prweb.com.
8. Quoted in John Gaudiosi, "How This Med School Is Using Virtual Reality to Teach Students," *Fortune*, October 16, 2015. http://fortune.com.
9. Quoted in Jo Best, "HoloLens, MD: Why This Medical School Will Teach Doctors Anatomy with Microsoft's Augmented Reality, Not Cadavers," ZDNet, December 14, 2016. www.zd net.com.
10. Quoted in CBS News, "From Virtual Reality to Medical Reality."

11. Quoted in CBS News, "From Virtual Reality to Medical Reality."

12. Quoted in Kate McGillivray, "Montreal-Made Virtual Reality Simulator Trains Young Surgeons," CBC News, January 7, 2016. www.cbc.ca.

13. Quoted in MobiHealthNews, "15 Health and Wellness Use Cases for Virtual Reality," June 22, 2017. www.mobihealth news.com.

14. Quoted in Mandy Erickson, "Virtual Reality System Helps Surgeons, Reassures Patients," Stanford Medicine, July 11, 2017. https://med.stanford.edu.

15. Quoted in CBS News, "Latest Tools for Neurosurgeons: Virtual Reality Headsets," May 4, 2015. www.cbsnews.com.

16. Quoted in CBS News, "Latest Tools for Neurosurgeons."

17. Quoted in CBS News, "Latest Tools for Neurosurgeons."

18. Quoted in Salix Pharmaceuticals, "Salix Pharmaceuticals Unveils 360-Degree Virtual Reality Experience to Evolve Medical Understanding About Irritable Bowel Syndrome," PR Newswire, May 3, 2017. www.prnewswire.com.

19. Quoted in Rebecca Hills-Duty, "Paramedics in Florida Using VR for Training," VRFocus, May 10, 2017. www.vrfocus.com.

20. Quoted in GetEducated.com, "Nursing Degrees Online Use Second Life Virtual Reality for Teaching," 2017. www.get educated.com.

21. Quoted in Gaudiosi, "How This Med School Is Using Virtual Reality to Teach Students."

Chapter 3: Studying and Treating the Brain

22. Quote in Billy Steele, "Patient Wears Headset to Map Brain During Surgery," *Engadget* (blog), February 17, 2016. www .engadget.com.

23. Quoted in Tina Amirtha, "Welcome to Brain Science's Next Frontier: Virtual Reality," *Fast Company*, November 19, 2015. www.fastcompany.com.

24. Quoted in Stuart Wolpert, "Brain's Reaction to Virtual Reality Should Prompt Further Study, Suggests New Research by UCLA Neuroscientists," UCLA Newsroom, November 24, 2014. http://newsroom.ucla.edu.

25. Quoted in MobiHealthNews, "15 Health and Wellness Use Cases for Virtual Reality."
26. Quoted in University of Texas at Dallas, "Virtual Reality Helps Children on Autism Spectrum Improve Social Skills," September 22, 2016. www.utdallas.edu.
27. Quoted in University of Texas at Dallas, "Virtual Reality Helps Children on Autism Spectrum Improve Social Skills."
28. Quoted in University of Texas at Dallas, "Virtual Reality Helps Children on Autism Spectrum Improve Social Skills."
29. Denise T. Reid, "Benefits of a Virtual Play Rehabilitation Environment for Children with Cerebral Palsy Perceptions of Self-Efficacy: A Pilot Study," *Pediatric Rehabilitation*, 2002. www .clinicasentidos.com.br/projeto/clinica-sentidos/arquivos /Benets_of_a_virtual_play_rehabilitation.pdf.
30. Quoted in Elizabeth Balboa, "Healthcare Professionals Pilot VR, AR-Based Therapies," Benzinga, August 7, 2017. www .benzinga.com.
31. Mona Lalwani, "GE's Neuro VR Experience Takes You Inside a Musician's Brain." EnGadget. August 6, 2015. www.engadget .com.

Chapter 4: Easing Pain and Anxiety

32. Quoted in McGoogan and Murgia, "Watch the World's First Surgery Streamed in Virtual Reality Live from London."
33. Quoted in Cade Metz, "A New Way for Therapists to Get Inside Heads: Virtual Reality," *New York Times*, July 30, 2017. www.nytimes.com.
34. Skip Rizzo, interview with author, August 14, 2017.
35. Rizzo, interview.
36. Rizzo, interview.
37. Rizzo, interview.
38. Quoted in Jo Marchant, "Virtually Painless—How VR Is Making Surgery Simpler," *Mosaic*, January 31, 2017. https://mosaic science.com.
39. Quoted in Rachel Metz, "Better than Opioids? Virtual Reality Could Be Your Next Painkiller," *MIT Technology Review*, July 18, 2016. www.technologyreview.com.
40. Rizzo, interview.

41. Rizzo, interview.
42. Quoted in Dana Guth, "Tufts Medical Center to Help Calm Anxiety with Virtual Reality," *Boston Wellness* (blog), *Boston Magazine*, December 7, 2015. www.bostonmagazine.com.
43. Quoted in Guth, "Tufts Medical Center to Help Calm Anxiety with Virtual Reality."
44. Quoted in Erickson, "Virtual Reality System Helps Surgeons, Reassures Patients."

Chapter 5: Easing the Challenges of Recovery
45. Rizzo, interview.
46. Rizzo, interview.
47. Quoted in Dean Takahashi, "VRPhysio Enables Patients to Do Physical Therapy in Virtual Reality," VentureBeat, April 2, 2017. https://venturebeat.com.
48. Quoted in Shakira Sanchez-Collins, "Virtual Reality and Exoskeleton Help Paraplegics Partially Recover, Study Finds," ABC News, August 11, 2016. http://abcnews.go.com.
49. Quoted in Aalborg University, "Virtual Reality Eases Phantom Limb Pain," ScienceDaily, May 31, 2017. www.sciencedaily.com.
50. Quoted in Aalborg University, "Virtual Reality Eases Phantom Limb Pain."
51. Rizzo, interview.

Books

Matthias Harders and Robert Riener, *Virtual Reality in Medicine*. New York: Springer, 2012.

Jason Jerald, *The VR Book: Human-Centered Design for Virtual Reality*. Williston, VT: Morgan and Claypool, 2015.

Jaron Lanier, *Dawn of the New Everything.* New York: Holt, 2017.

Tony Parisi, *Learning Virtual Reality*. Sebastopol, CA: O'Reilly Media, 2015.

Murray Ramirez, *Virtual Reality for Beginners: How to Understand, Use & Create with VR*. Seattle, WA: CreateSpace, 2016.

Internet Sources

Erin Carson, "10 Ways Virtual Reality Is Revolutionizing Medicine and Healthcare," TechRepublic, April 8, 2015. www.techrepublic.com.

Daniel Freeman and Jason Freeman, "How Virtual Reality Could Transform Mental Health Treatment," *Know Your Mind* (blog), *Psychology Today*, May 13, 2016. www.psychologytoday.com.

VR Today Magazine, "Top 6 Incredible Uses of Medical Virtual Reality," May 13, 2017. https://vrtodaymagazine.com.

Websites

USC Institute for Creative Technologies: Medical Virtual Reality (http://medvr.ict.usc.edu). This site reveals the many innovations being made at one of the top institutions making remarkable strides treating mental and physical disorders with VR.

Virtual Reality Society (www.vrs.org.uk). This British-based site keeps track of the latest news in VR, as well as new apps, profiles of innovators, and the many ways VR is being used in medicine, science, entertainment, and more.

VR Medicine News (www.vrmedicinenews.com). This site provides the latest news on how virtual reality is being used in patient care, medical training, and in other aspects of health care and research from around the world.

Western University of Health Sciences J and K Virtual Reality Learning Center (www.westernu.edu/virtualrealitylearningcenter). See how medical students at Western University are using the latest in VR to learn about anatomy, surgery, veterinary medicine, physical therapy, and many other branches of health care.

INDEX

PICTURE CREDITS

James Roland started out as a newspaper reporter more than twenty-five years ago and then moved on to become an editor, magazine writer, and author.